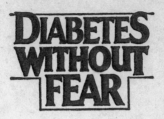

DIABETES WITHOUT FEAR

Dr. Joseph I. Goodman

"Refreshing...a distillation of many years of practice
and bedside experience...the positive and optimistic
approach to diabetes."

> Max Ellenburg, M.D., past president of
> the American Diabetes Association

"I recommend this book with enthusiasm."

> Henry Dolger, M.D.,
> past Chief of Diabetes Clinic;
> Mt. Sinai Hospital, New York

DIABETES WITHOUT FEAR

Dr. Joseph I. Goodman
with W. Watts Biggers

AVON BOOKS ◆ NEW YORK

The authors gratefully acknowledge permission to include material from the following:

From "A Dialogue about Diabetes and Exercise" by E.A. and D.F. Sims. Reprinted from *Diabetes Forecast,* Copyright © 1974 by permission of the American Diabetes Association.

From "Juvenile Diabetes: A Tragic Difference in Children" by B. Vincent, *The Cleveland Press,* May 22, 1974. Copyright © 1974. By permission of *The Cleveland Press.*

From "Life With Diabetes" by L. Matthews and E. Hill, *Diabetes Newsletter,* Diabetes Association of Greater Cleveland, 2022 Lee Road, Cleveland, Ohio 44118, April, 1974. By permission of *Diabetes Newsletter.*

From "Ron Santo and Diabetes: Accepted It, Live a Full Life" by J. Shaw. Reprinted from *Sportsmedicine* Magazine, June 1974 by permsiion of the publisher, McGraw-Hill, Inc.

CONTENTS

FOREWORD

I BELIEVE THE value of this book has already been proven. Through an odd twist of fate, it was proven even before the publisher received the complete manuscript. Let me explain.

When Dr. Goodman asked me to work on *Diabetes Without Fear* to help make the material more readily understandable to readers unfamiliar with medical terminology and concepts, I clearly saw the need for such a book, but I saw it only from an intellectual viewpoint. Because no one in my immediate family had diabetes, I was not emotionally involved.

Then, about halfway through my work on the book, my wife Grace was rushed to the hospital with internal bleeding—completely without warning. For many weeks, Grace went through one crisis after another, the entire episode finally culminating in major vascular surgery.

The operation was a dramatic success. But our doctors had one piece of bad news: Grace had diabetes.

I shall never forget the day the doctors made that announcement—the dual shock I felt, the strange look which came into Grace's eyes (she knew, of course, that I was working on *Diabetes Without Fear*); nor will I ever forget what Dr. Goodman's book meant to Grace and to me as we coped with the knowledge that she was a diabetic.

I know both of us well enough to be fully aware of the unwarranted fears, the complex exaggerations that would almost certainly have clouded our vision. But thanks to *Diabetes Without Fear* (I had the whole book in my head!), we were able to meet every challenge, quickly put to rest any trepidations, counteract the many half-truths we had read or seen on television and politely ignore all that "advice" from neighbors, friends and relatives.

Diabetes Without Fear has been and continues to be a blessing for our lives. I hope it will be the same for yours.

W. WATTS BIGGERS

1

FICTION
VERSUS FACT

"THE MOST AMAZING thing about diabetes is the complete lack of true knowledge that exists about it," says Mary Tyler Moore. "When I first learned I had it, I was very frightened. I wondered, 'Am I going to be an invalid? Will I be bedridden?' I just didn't know."

Unfortunately, the actress' experience is not unusual. Diabetes is probably the most misunderstood of all diseases—so much so that by the time the majority of my patients come to consult me for advice on the management of their diabetes, they have already developed emotionally crippling inhibitions which prevent them from enjoying the normal existence that should be theirs.

The news that one has an incurable disease—*any* incurable disease—is traumatic in itself, and in the case of diabetes, what the typical patient knows of the disease serves only to magnify the trauma. Thanks to pseudo-scientific books, so-called "documentaries" on television and old wives' tales, the newly diagnosed patient quickly develops a swarm of unrealistic fears about diabetes. He connects the disease with visions of physical deterioration, gangrene, amputation, blindness, dangerous complications, shock from too much insulin and coma from too *little* insulin; he worries that he will lose his job, that he can never have children, that he should never marry; he becomes frustrated by the thought of diet restrictions and the inability to have sugar or alcohol ever again. The list of frightening apparitions is endless.

Aside from the terrible toll such unnecessary fears take on the patients themselves, imagine what they do to members of the diabetic's family. Husbands and wives of diabetics wonder if their marriages can ever be "normal" again. Brothers and sisters of diabetics, often neglected in favor of the overprotected diabetic child, are forced into confused, guilt-ridden existences. Children of diabetics develop unhealthy eating habits and doubts about their own futures. Parents of diabetics often feel plagued by gnawing guilt and blame themselves for their child's fate, doubting their ability to cope with the future.

"I honestly wasn't too upset when they first told me my son had it," said Keith, a hospital worker. "I'd seen lots of diabetics in my job. But then I remembered this TV story—a police show—about a diabetic who went into coma just because he accidentally took too much insulin without eating. And then I remembered I'd heard the same kind of thing from a neighbor, about how her nephew died with it. And I got to wondering what it was going to be like worrying every day about being certain we did everything just right for my son or else that would happen to him. All of a sudden I didn't think I could handle it. I started to fall apart."

Millions of other diabetics and their families similarly fall apart, not because of the reality of their disease, but because of their unfounded fears about what they *believe* the disease is like and what it will do to them. I have invented a term for this dangerous emotional disturbance—"diabetic neurosis." It is a vicious neurosis, often more destructive than the disease itself, and it begins the moment the patient is told that he has diabetes. Why?

First of all, few people are prepared when they discover they have the disease. Although untreated diabetes has very recognizable symptoms—frequent urination, excessive thirst, insatiable hunger, weight loss, fatigue—most determinations are made well before such symptoms become severe; usually it is by chance, during a routine medical checkup by the patient's doctor, or in a hospital where the patient has been admitted for some other disorder or even during a preemployment or insurance examination.

Having had no previous suggestion of the illness, the typical patient is armed with nothing but hearsay. Imagine, then, his reaction to the announcement that he has diabetes.

"It was like a building fell on me," Brian, a jewelry salesman in his mid-thirties, told me. "I've always been an active guy, and when the insurance doc told me I had diabetes, it seemed like a dead end for my whole life. Maybe I didn't know too much about it, but what I did know was all bad."

Brian had always prided himself on his sound physical condition. He was an avid jogger. "When they told me about the diabetes, right away I thought about a book I'd read—this story about a guy who lost his legs—and that made me think about my own legs. I remember reaching down to touch them and wondering if the next thing would be they'll have to chop them off."

Fear of "complications" is one of the primary causes of diabetic neurosis—such fear may even produce physical illness with no physiological connection to diabetes. "I keep worrying about what my condition will lead to," a dental receptionist told me. "I've heard things, you know, insulin shock and all that. From the minute they told me I had the disease, I've been worrying so much I can't sleep right. And I'm afraid to take anything to make me sleep. My boss says that might not mix with insulin. So I'm becoming a nervous wreck.

My doctor says if I don't calm myself, I'm a prime candidate for ulcers."

The problem of the patient's lack of accurate information is often compounded by the physician. In the case of a twenty-one-year-old college student named Mary, her gynecologist, discovering her diabetes in the course of a routine examination, immediately sat her down and volunteered this advice:

"Since you have diabetes, you must carefully weigh the problems of marriage. You probably can't conceive. And if you do, there are all the dangers associated with pregnancy in diabetes—acidosis, hypertension and so on. If you should manage to overcome these hazards, the baby probably will not live or, if so, will be afflicted with congenital deformities."

An incredible diagnosis of the situation, totally untrue! Luckily, Mary was a very levelheaded young woman. When she came to me, we were able to reapproach the subject, wipe away this misinformation and send her on to a happy, well-rounded life. But imagine the psychological damage which might have been done to a less stable personality—one like twenty-three-year-old Darlene, for example.

This young woman was so fearful and guilt-ridden about her future that she insisted on attempting to cure herself through "faith in God." Although her pastor and his wife, as well as her doctor, sought desperately to dissuade her from attempting this "faith cure," the distraught young woman persisted. After three days without insulin, she lapsed into a coma and needlessly, tragically died.

Consider the case of David, the diabetic son of actress Dina Merrill. Ms. Merrill explains why diabetic neurosis was responsible for her son's death: "He was sure that his life would be short, or interfered with by blindness or something because of the diabetes, so he wanted instant results with everything, wanted to pack as much living in while he could. Always it was speed, speed, speed. Fast cars, fast boats. That's what killed him."

David died in a high-speed motorboat accident just ten days short of his twenty-fourth birthday.

But even this was not the end of his story, as far as diabetic neurosis was concerned. Convinced that diabetes was hereditary, Dina Merrill guiltily researched her family tree. "We've checked back on both sides of the family, but we haven't found it yet. Evidently it can skip five or six generations."

The truth is, there is no reliable evidence proving that diabetes is hereditary at all!

Misinformation, then, is the chief cause of diabetic neurosis, a situation which is only worsened by most of the current literature.

"The more I read," says Brian, "the worse it got. Diabetes sounded like the first step toward everything bad. Right away, you're stopped from eating and drinking anything you want, but that doesn't guarantee a thing. You don't live any longer. It just *seems* longer. If you go out and cut your foot, you may lose it. And if you just sit in a chair and watch TV, you'll probably go blind."

It's not difficult to locate some of the possible sources of Brian's misinformation. The following statement was made by no less than a president of the American Diabetes Association and given wide dissemination in the *Wall Street Journal*[1]:

"Nearly all diabetics eventually develop degenerative complications resulting from premature hardening of the arteries and deterioration of the body's kidneys. Diabetes has just become the country's leading cause of new cases of blindness. The vascular complications shorten the average diabetic's life by one-third; a child is lucky to live twenty-five or thirty years after the onset of the illness. Their lives still are short and troubled. Because the complications rather than the disease often appear on death certificates, statistics hide diabetes' role as the United States' second leading cause of death."

This type of desperately unbalanced statement, although made for a good cause such as the solicitation of funds for research, clearly does more harm than good. Imagine the mental anguish of the newly diagnosed diabetic or a member of the family—or, for that matter, even a diabetic who has had the disease for many years—reading such a statement.

Linda is an example. This is the letter she wrote to a very prestigious magazine after reading its special issue devoted to the "future" for diabetics: "I was terrified by your special issue. My own doctor tells me that I don't have anything to worry about with my eyes even after eighteen years of diabetes, yet your magazine says that most diabetics are going to lose their sight! What can I do to prevent this? What are my chances of going blind?"[2]

And what about this from a recent newspaper?

"Diabetes is one of the most underrated of all major killers, including cancer, heart and kidney disease. It's not a disease that can be cured. In fact, it's not even a disease, but a genetic malfunction of the pancreas that inevitably affects the entire body. It is a serious ailment in itself, and is more serious because it is a contributing factor in a host of other disabling illnesses. It is thought to be the leading cause of new cases of blindness and gangrene amputations, half of all heart attacks, three-fourths of all strokes and the underlying source of the majority of uremia (kidney poisoning) cases. It therefore constitutes a major health threat."[3]

This picture is pessimistic, depressing—and totally misleading. Although the effects of diabetes obviously can be serious, and should not be minimized, the important fact is that the great majority of diabetics lead healthy, active lives; that persons who have had diabetes for twenty, thirty, forty, even fifty years can function quite normally; that today there are television and movie stars, high government officials, even professional sports figures with diabetes who lead full, highly successful lives without a hint of abnormality. In fact, because they take better care of themselves, their lives are perhaps longer and healthier than if they had *not* had diabetes.

In the view of the medical profession, diabetes cannot be ranked with heart disease and cancer as a leading killer. Most doctors are inclined to view diabetes as a more or less benign process. In fact, Dr. L. Matthews of Case Western Reserve University writes, "I've had diabetes since 1957 . . . [and] if one *has* to have a chronic disease, and we really have no choice, then I feel we are fortunate to have diabetes!"[4]

But the diabetic knows none of this. Everything he reads or hears about his condition is presented from the kind of pessimistic viewpoint which causes him to wonder, "Am I finished? Can I get married? Should I have children? Will I soon become too weak to hold a job?"

And while questions such as these are bombarding him, the diabetic can expect to be arbitrarily denied life and health insurance, rejected by misguided potential employers, even thwarted in his application for a driver's license.

The vice-president of a large corporation was anxious to hire a very talented young woman who was one of my patients. During the pre-employment examination, the company physician discovered that the applicant was a diabetic and stated, "Your sugar is high. I'll have to reject you." Despite the recommendation—a very strong one—from a company officer, the doctor refused my patient, labeling her as unsuitable for employment. Imagine what this did to the patient's sense of purpose and self-confidence, and what a waste of talent it was—all due to private and professional ignorance about the true nature of diabetes.

When race car driver Dick Batchelder learned in 1973 that he had diabetes, one of the first things he recalled was someone once telling him that diabetics could not get a license to drive. "I thought of that and wondered, 'What happens to me now? What about my job, my family, my racing career?'"

It was an oppressive fear of a type he had never known before. It almost conquered him—but he managed to break free and that same year went on to set a new track record in the Canadian American Classic at Star Speedway in New Hampshire.

There are hundreds of success stories like this. Consider only these few: Carol Channing, hockey star Bobby Clarke, actress Gail Patrick, George Jessel, baseball star Ron Santo, Dan Rowan, former tennis star Bill Talbert. So why are there so many depressing words written about diabetes?

If blindness is only a sometime result of diabetes, why do so many articles, books and TV shows imply that it is almost inevitable?

If candy, cake and alcohol need not be dropped from the diabetic's diet, why do most written materials state the opposite?

If diabetic parents need not live in fear that their children are certain to be diabetic too, why aren't they told this?

If the use of insulin can be simple and safe, why should TV stories imply the opposite?

Why, in short, have almost one hundred percent of diabetic writings focused on the most negative aspects of the disease? Certainly, much of what is being disseminated *was* once true—but is true no longer. Certainly, too, there is far more drama, far more sales appeal in a story which builds to tragedy—to gangrene, amputation, divorce, blindness, frustration, coma, death —than one in which all ends well. Perhaps those doing the writing have been so concerned with the importance of following prescribed treatment that they have neglected the positive aspects of diabetes.

Regardless of the reason, the fact is that nothing of significance has been written about the great strides medicine has made in understanding diabetes and in helping patients live with it easily, safely and comfortably. And, tragically, this vacuum, combined with a growing mountain of misinformation, has served only to insure that diabetics and their families will suffer from diabetic neurosis. It is a mountain I have had to confront again and again throughout my more than forty years as a diabetes specialist, both in private and hospital practice.

Today, there are an estimated ten million Americans who have diabetes, and, conservatively, another thirty million whose lives are intimately intertwined with one or more diabetic. Thus, some twenty percent of this nation's total population is affected by a myriad of totally unnecessary emotional disturbances connected with this disease. This makes diabetic neurosis one of the most serious health problems facing our country.

In this book, the various fears and anxieties which preoccupy the diabetic and his family are discussed, frequently in the patients' own words, and the background of their emotional reactions analyzed in some detail. I have undertaken to counteract these disturbing factors in much the same way that I do in my private practice: All sides of the problem under discussion are presented from a rational scientific standpoint, with realities, sound, practical advice and how-to information substituted for exaggerations and half-truths. In this way, the patient and members of his family will be able to view the situation with reassurance and optimism—and hope for a normal life.

2

BASIC QUESTIONS
AND ANSWERS

IF IGNORANCE and misinformation are the basis for diabetic neurosis, then education is obviously the key to prevention and cure. But what kind of education? How much? And how should it be obtained ?

"I honestly think my doctor's attitude changed toward me the minute he found out I had diabetes," a thirty-five-year-old computer operator told me. "He always took plenty of time with me before, but when I got diabetes, he just handed me a pamphlet from some clinic and told me to talk with his nurse."

How much time should the doctor himself spend explaining the nature and treatment of diabetes? Physicians sometimes turn their patients over to nurses and dieticians or even other diabetics, but this is not necessarily the best possible schooling. There is, after all, a great deal that is new and very meaningful for the diabetic and the family to learn. Most of it may seem quite simple to a thoroughly trained physician, but not to the patient and his family.

"More than anything else, it's the needle that frightens me," a young mother told me. "I'm always afraid it will break off while I'm giving myself the shot, so I hate the idea of being alone when I do it. And yet I don't like my husband or my children—especially my children—watching me. So I keep on doing it alone, even though I'm terrified."

Fear of the needle breaking is only one of many

18

expressed to me by patients who have not been properly educated about diabetes. Typical questions are:

What about air bubbles? Is it true they can kill?

Will my arms and legs become unsightly in the places where the needles are constantly used?

Would there be less chance of this if I had fewer shots per day?

If some of the insulin runs out, should I try to give myself a small second shot, or could that be dangerous?

Are some insulins better than others?

Is there danger in exercising? Should I stop my son from participating in school sports?

It is time to offer some answers.

Who should educate?

From the moment diabetes is diagnosed, both the patient and his family should enter a learning process sufficient not only to dispel the rumors, myths and distortions associated with diabetes, but also to make the diabetic's "tools"—his diet, oral drugs, insulin and needles—as familiar and friendly as the controls of an automobile to a skilled driver.

The new diabetic requires a bare minimum of twelve hours of individual instruction, but some physicians, perhaps considering themselves poor communicators or feeling they cannot economically devote this amount of time to the disease, seek other methods for educating their patients.

Dr. B. R. Boshell, for example, maintains that other diabetics are the best teachers for new diabetic patients and, therefore, turns over much of the responsibility for instruction to them.[1] In this way, patients are taught how to walk into any restaurant and estimate food exchanges, how to alter dosages of insulin and how to make urine tests. This instruction is sup-

plemented by written material including a handbook
and an individualized "blue book" containing the patient's medication schedule and all tests from his first
day of admission. There is also a "yellow book" for
permanent recording of four-times-daily blood and
urine sugar tests in the hospital and, later, at home.

Despite these materials, however, I consider the
process ineffective and even dangerous. First, the lack
of formal training for such "teachers" tends to lower
the level of importance attached to this education by
the new diabetic. If it were really important, they are
inclined to think, my doctor would be doing this for
me. Second, the patient-teachers may well be asked to
respond to questions for which they are not properly
prepared. Third, any errors these patient-teachers may
themselves have picked up will be passed along and
very likely compounded by their pupils.

Recognizing these dangers, some doctors have turned
to courses offered by hospital-established units of
specially trained personnel, such as nurses and dieticians, to instruct new patients in their diabetic care.
But here again there are intrinsic weaknesses. Consider the results of such a course offered at the E. J.
Meyer Memorial Hospital in Buffalo, New York. Immediately following the course, the new patients appeared highly proficient at techniques such as insulin
injection, but only three months later, both their general knowledge of the disease and their proficiency at
self-care had declined decisively. Moreover, their course
suffered a tremendously high dropout rate—of the
original forty-six patients, only nine remained to complete the instruction.[2]

The dropout rate was less when offered to a second
group, of clinic outpatients this time; however, at the
end of the program, the best they could do on questions designed to test their knowledge of the management of diabetes was an average of fifty-five percent
correct. They had poor knowledge of meal planning

and proper diet, and little idea of how to properly test for acetone in the urine.

Clearly, doctor substitutes are often unsuccessful in the education of patients, and this is not surprising. What is too often overlooked or ignored is the fact that with diabetes, unlike most other diseases, education is not a subordinate matter in terms of patient health; rather, it is a major part of the "treatment." As such, it demands the physician's personal attention. Only in this way will the patient attach sufficient importance to the matter to listen and learn to the best of his or her ability, to stay until the "course" is complete and to receive the kind of answers the questions deserve.

What is diabetes?

The full name is Diabetes Mellitus, and the disease results when the beta cells of the pancreas fail to provide a sufficient supply of effective insulin. Without this hormone, the body is unable to change foods—proteins, fats, carbohydrates—into the energy needed to sustain life and keep the body functioning properly. We do not know why this occurs—why the pancreas ceases to fulfill its insulin function—but age and overweight often play a role.

There is no known cure for diabetes, but it can be controlled in one of three ways:

1. Diet alone.
2. Oral medication.
3. Insulin.

Insulin

"What is insulin?"

On January 11, 1922, Drs. Frederick Banting and Charles Best injected an extract from an animal pancreas into a teenager, Leonard Thompson, who lay gravely ill with diabetes. Almost immediately, Thompson improved, and within days after being on the verge of death, the seventy-five-pounder had dramatically regained his weight and strength.

And so the world hailed the discovery of the extract, insulin, the first effective means of treating diabetes. It was a medical miracle, a momentous discovery which eventually won a Nobel Prize for Drs. Banting and Best—there is no way to overestimate its importance. Without it, a book such as this one would be impossible, for there would be little to discuss on the positive side of diabetes for the millions who can now look forward to a happy, normal life.

Today, more than fifty years after Banting and Best's discovery, physicians have a wide variety of insulins to choose from for their patients, depending upon how long they wish the preparation to continue acting. The original product produced by Banting and Best, regular insulin, works for a relatively short time, and it was primarily in order to prolong this period that other insulins were developed.

The following summary of types and technical names will demonstrate the variety of preparations available. Bear in mind that although various types are grouped together, no substitutions in any patient's program should be made without his physician's approval.

1. Short or rapid-acting.
   a. *Regular*
   b. *Semi-lente*
2. Intermediate-acting.
   a. *Globin*
   b. *NPH (Isophane)*
   c. *Lente*
3. Long-acting.
   a. *Protamine Zinc*
   b. *Ultra-lente*

"What about the different numbers on insulin? My druggist was out of U-100 and offered to sell me U-80. I said no and went elsewhere, but it left me wondering."

Unless they have been given a thorough grounding in the diabetic "tools," this is an area almost certain to confuse patient and family alike. In the case in question, the patient used better judgment than the druggist. Although, in theory, there is no reason why a patient using U-100 insulin could not substitute U-80, the danger lies in possible miscalculation of the patient's prescribed dosage.

The rule is to keep sufficient insulin of the proper concentration on hand (always one bottle in reserve) so that if your druggist is out of what you need, there is ample time for him to order or to shop at another drugstore. For those who wish to understand the differences between the various concentrations of insulin, however, let me explain.

Insulins are sold in three main concentrations: U-40 (red label), U-80 (green label) and U-100 (black label). The difference is in how much liquid volume the preparation contains for each unit of insulin—or, to look at it another way, how "pure" the preparation is in terms of insulin. With U-100 preparations, a single cc of the liquid contains 100 units of insulin, while with U-80, that same amount of liquid contains only 80 units of insulin, and with U-40, only 40 units. Thus, you have to inject twice as much U-40 to get the same amount of insulin as with U-80.

Over the years, there has been much confusion because of the different concentrations. Insulin syringes were marked with two scales so that they could be used with either U-40 or U-80 insulin, and as a result patients were mistakenly using the wrong scale and injecting themselves with half, or, much worse, twice their prescribed dosage. The result in the latter case was insulin shock.

Today, U-40 and U-80 syringes and insulin preparations are being phased out slowly and U-100 disposable and reusable syringes, capable of accurately delivering all dosages needed, are being used much more widely. The exclusive use of U-100 insulin should greatly reduce patient confusion, especially because of its compatibility with our decimal system. There is no danger in a doctor shifting his patient to the highly purified U-100 product. No actual change in insulin dosage is required, just a reduction in liquid volume, and control is unaffected. If a patient is in good control before the change, he or she should remain in good control afterward.[8]

For the U-100 concentrations of insulin, the four syringes currently available are: the 1 cc (100 units) disposable syringe, the 1 cc (100 units) glass syringe, the .50 cc (50 units) disposable syringe and the .35 cc (35 units) glass syringe.

All of these syringes are simple to operate and extremely well-made. Fears of needles bending or breaking are totally without foundation. In all my years of practice, I have never had this happen to one of my patients.

"It's an awful problem keeping my insulin refrigerated when I go for a visit overnight. Is there any simple way to handle this?"

There certainly is: Forget it. All the complicated methods used by diabetics to insure refrigeration are totally unnecessary. I have talked to patients who carried ice or used special thermos bottles or other cold devices wherever they traveled for more than a day, but the truth of the matter is that insulin being used by the patient does not deteriorate at room temperature and thus does not need refrigeration.

"I worry about air bubbles in the syringe. How dangerous are they? And if a bubble makes me lose any of the insulin, should I give myself a small second shot?"

Questions like this one (and they are quite common) again point up the importance of proper patient education. A colleague of mine told me of a recently diagnosed diabetic who accidentally injected himself with a whole vial of air. Recognizing what he had done, the patient called for an ambulance and then lay down, prepared to die.

Actually, there is no danger from air—whether a whole vial or a single bubble—unless it is injected directly into a vein. Air in the syringe is to be avoided because of this possibility, but the properly informed patient knows how unlikely this is, especially since he is trained how to give injections in a manner which avoids the veins.

As for giving additional insulin if some should be lost (for whatever reason), the answer is an emphatic no. If the amount is relatively small, the loss may be ignored. If it is more than a single unit or two, the patient's physician should be consulted.

"A woman who lived in the neighborhood where I grew up had diabetes. She used to talk to my mother about it, and I will never forget those ugly, scooped-out places on her upper arms. I've been worried about this from the first minute they told me what I have. I guess I'll have to get rid of all my short-sleeved blouses, won't I?"

This attractive young woman's fears were groundless. The condition she referred to, *lipoatrophy*, never affected more than a relatively small percentage of diabetics at any time, and today even that number has been drastically reduced. Lipoatrophy—hollowed-out areas at the site of insulin injection—results from the disappearance of fat, and it is often preceded or accompanied by swelling (lipohypertrophy) in these same areas.

The cause of this was unknown until recently, and there was no specific treatment. Now, however, it is recognized that the condition is a reaction to certain material in insulin (non-insulin protein material and pro-insulin-like substances) which produce antibodies. In 1973, the highly purified insulin U-100 was introduced, and this has markedly decreased the number of patients who display allergic reactions which lead to lipoatrophy or lipohypertrophy. In fact, this new insulin has even been effective in revitalizing the sunken or swollen areas of patients who had previously displayed these conditions. Dr. S. M. Wentworth and his associates, at a meeting of the American Diabetes Association, reported improvement or complete disappearance of atrophy due to insulin lipoatrophy in eighty-five percent of the patients tested, and similar results were reported for insulin allergy by a team from the Lilly Laboratory for Clinical Research.[4]

One caution, however: Although this purer insulin, U-100, has greatly reduced the incidence of unsightly tissue conditions, the diabetic is still well-advised to rotate the site of insulin injections. Without such rotation, thickened skin may build up and make the giving of injections more difficult and discomforting.

Best insulin dosage

"If I have diabetes because I lack adequate insulin, and if I inject adequate insulin, why don't I become completely normal?"

The answer is that medical science to date is unable to match the function of the pancreas. In order to make the diabetic completely "normal," insulin would have to be made available to the body at the precise times and in the precise amounts that it would be released from the pancreas of the non-diabetic person. This cannot be done.

The diabetic whose pancreas is incapable of secreting sufficient insulin must rely on an injected product, one which is absorbed into the bloodstream at a uniform rate over several hours. The injected product cannot respond to body demands. For example, the regular rate of absorption will not increase because the patient decides to eat an especially heavy meal, nor will it decrease because the patient extends the hours between meals.

The simple truth is that, although insulin has been available for more than half a century, we are not yet skilled enough in its use to restore the blood sugar of the diabetic to absolute normal.[5] Although I am confident this day will come in the not too far distant future (see Chapter Eight), for the present the proper treatment for the diabetic is that program which best enables his body to most closely approximate insulin normalcy on a consistent basis.

"Once my doctor decided on the right dosage for my diabetes, why should he change it? I had been doing fine for two months, and all of a sudden he changed the amounts. Does that make sense?"

Indeed it does. Be thankful that your doctor watches you carefully and notes the signs which indicate a need for change. Patients and their families should prepare themselves for an ever-changing pattern in terms of insulin dosage. Why? Because the blood glucose of diabetic patients is characteristically variable. Wide swings from high levels to low levels and back again are commonplace. It is almost impossible to avoid such fluctuations even in the well-regulated diabetic.

The tragedy is that great numbers of patients, having "managed" their diabetes by way of a fixed insulin dose over a period of many years, now suffer with crippling disabilities. Their blood glucose levels have changed, but their insulin dosage has not.

There is no rule more important to the insulin-taking diabetic than this one: *Frequent reassessment of the insulin dose is essential.*

"This guy and I were patients together at the hospital, and I know for a fact my blood sugar was never higher than his, but he only has to take one injection a day now that he's home, and my doctor has me taking two. Can you think of any logical reason for that?"

I certainly can. The hospital environment and the home environment are quite different. Two patients might have quite similar blood sugar patterns while in the hospital and quite different ones at home. More importantly, patients should not complain about programs which require more than a single dose of insulin. Some of the most common errors of treatment occur when physicians attempt to maintain every diabetic on one dose of insulin daily.

A classic example is the one quoted by Dr. P. Forsham in connection with protamine zinc insulin. In 1946, the arrival of this long-acting insulin was hailed as a great breakthrough. In one sense, it was, but in another sense it was "the worst thing that ever could have happened to diabetes, because it failed to deliver the necessary big dose during peak body demand. Many juvenile diabetics who were on protamine zinc insulin exclusively for twenty years or more are now blind, sick and dying."[6] Even more tragic in Dr. Forsham's view (and mine) is the fact that he continues to see *new* patients who have been on protamine zinc for twenty years.

There is no single foolproof method of fitting a patient's insulin dosage to the fluctuations which occur in his blood glucose level. The Joslin Clinic uses two doses per day of intermediate and short-acting insulins. To this end, mixtures of lente and semi-lente and, occasionally, ultra-lente are used.

About a two-shot regimen versus those requiring only a single injection, Dr. Forsham says, "Patients unaccustomed to the two shots will complain at first but will soon feel so much better in the afternoon and evening that they will be happy to comply."

Some years ago, Dr. Robert Jackson treated a large group of juvenile diabetics very successfully at the University of Iowa, without complications, using *four* doses of regular insulin, morning, noon, dinner- and bedtime. When the doctor suggested that an intermediate insulin, globin, could be substituted before dinner to avoid waking the child for the late dose, the parents invariably asked, "Will my child get along as well on three doses of insulin as he has been doing on four?"

This is the attitude which should be adopted by all patients. The question put to the doctor should not be, "How many shots can I get by with?" Rather, it should be, "How many shots will provide the best possible management of my diabetes?"

Insulin reaction

What is hypoglycemia?

"Last week I had a horrible experience in school," an eighteen-year-old woman relates. "I knew something was wrong so I went to the principal's office. I told the assistant principal I was feeling funny and needed orange juice. He went to the refrigerator and brought me some. Before I could drink it, I passed out, grabbed him and started pulling at him. Why do I always get violent when I have an insulin reaction? I want to hurt people. I make a damn fool of myself. I have only three more days of school, but I know the kids are talking. What do you think they're saying? By the way, I have a scholarship to college. Thank goodness I'm going to live away from home. Why do I get violent?"[7]

In another case, that of a forty-five-year-old male,

frequent periods of hypoglycemia, often causing double vision, made his wife and daughter fearful of letting him out of their sight. This, in turn, symbolized invalidism to the husband and father, made him feel old and dependent, and this "loss of manhood" led to severe depression.

How is the diabetic to cope with hypoglycemia?

The normal function of the brain is dependent on an adequate supply of glucose and oxygen. If the blood glucose level is allowed to become unduly low, the brain is unable to carry out its normal activity. Should this condition remain unchecked, the concentration of glucose dropping below critical levels, a number of very unpleasant symptoms can occur.

The earliest of these result from the effect of low blood glucose on the sympathetic nervous system and may include:

A rapid heart rate, pounding pulse, excessive perspiration, headache, hunger, pallor, nervousness, trembling, acute anxiety, abdominal pain, nausea, vomiting (on rare occasions) and blurred vision.

If these first symptoms, the body's "early warning system," go unheeded, a second set of symptoms may develop. These include:

Hyperexcitability, irritability, poor coordination, inability to concentrate, drowsiness, fatigue, confusion, inappropriate behavior, crying, loss of consciousness and generalized convulsions.

Such a listing of symptoms makes it clear that the violent conduct of the high school girl was not exceptional in the case of hypoglycemia. The important point to bear in mind here is that forewarned should mean forearmed. With proper care and preparation, such symptoms should never develop, and, if they do, can be counteracted in a matter of minutes or seconds.

Toward this end, schoolteachers and officers should be given a thorough understanding of the symptoms, signs and treatment of insulin reactions which may occur during school hours. Moreover, all diabetics, children and adults alike, should carry with them some source of sugar—honey or corn syrup or some type of candy—which can be consumed at the first sign of insulin reaction.

A rapid, very neat way to treat such reactions, if available in your area, is Instant Glucose. This thick, syrupy jelly is packaged in a collapsible tube for easy administration and a generous squeeze releases the concentrated glucose into the patient's mouth. It is absorbed rapidly, and the hypoglycemia is overcome within fifteen to twenty minutes. Instant Glucose was developed by Dr. Jack Leonards of Western Reserve University and is available through the Diabetes Association of Greater Cleveland, Ohio.

In the normal (non-diabetic) body, insulin secretion is regulated so that only the amount required at the moment is released from the pancreas. When no longer needed, the flow of insulin into the bloodstream is shut off. By contrast, the insulin administered to diabetic patients is not subject to the controls of the pancreas. The insulin dose is injected into the subcutaneous space (the space beneath the skin) where it remains until it is consumed, and during this period the insulin is absorbed into the bloodstream at a fixed rate. There is no shutoff valve. The insulin continues to lower the blood sugar even between meals when the patient is without food. It is this situation which, if not understood and taken into account, can lead to hypoglycemia—when, for example, the patient's insulin dosage is based on the expectation of "snacking" every two hours and the snack is ignored or, worse, an entire meal is skipped.

Patients on low-calorie reducing diets are particularly prone to hypoglycemia unless extreme care is taken to reassess their insulin dosage on a regular basis. Many such overweight patients experience a complete reversal of their diabetes when they begin taking a low-calorie diet—often to such a degree as to cause them to wonder if they ever had the disease. Obviously, a greatly reduced regimen of insulin is called for in patients on reducing diets. When the low-calorie diet is first put into effect, insulin requirements may be lowered by as much as fifty percent.

Another common cause of insulin reaction is a more-than-usual amount of exercise. No diabetic, young or old, needs to give up normal exercise or sports activity. He or she need only be properly prepared for what this exercise will demand. Physical activity revs up the body metabolism, causing blood glucose to be consumed by the body at a more rapid rate, while the insulin continues to be absorbed by the body at the normal rate. The effect of this situation is graphically expressed by Dorothea Sims:

"Early in my diabetes, I remember the sense of injustice with which I gulped orange juice laced with sugar during an insulin reaction which followed the unplanned-for and unrecognized exercise of running up- and downstairs looking after the children when they were all sick at once. I soon learned at a very basic level that, with my type of diabetes, I need to carry some form of sugar available on me at all times, even in the most apparently routine situations such as cleaning house, or shoveling snow, or mowing the lawn.

"Of course, this applies as well to the time when we plan a hike, a swim or a bike ride, or when I work in our vegetable garden. In these circumstances, I not only carry carbohydrate in some form with me, as well as my small insulin travel kit, but I always eat somewhat more than my usual intake at the meal before we begin, with emphasis on protein for its staying power —for example, an extra glass of milk and a cracker with peanut butter and jelly. I find that I need to supplement the meal with sugar about every twenty to thirty minutes when hiking or cross-country skiing.

"In spite of years of experience, there are still pitfalls for me. The commonest mistake is for me to forget to replenish the store of candy in my purse, parka or suitcase. If I am especially happy in some form of exercise, I sometimes forget to keep track of time. In general, I find that I have developed a kind of reflex yet subconscious method of evaluating all the elements in any given situation in order to stay up-to-date with the changing scene.

"In my own head, I compare it to the skill with which we drive our cars, habitual enough so that it is not a distraction from work or play, and yet alert and calculating enough to respond to signs of imbalance."[8]

Ms. Sims is entirely correct. Diabetics, especially as they become more familiar with the signs and symptoms of their disease, need have no fear of hypoglycemia if they adhere to these few relatively simple rules:

1. Take special precautions with low-calorie diets; discuss the diet change in detail with your physician.
2. When more than the usual amount of exercise is anticipated and the usual dosage of insulin injected, additional food must be consumed during and for several hours following the exercise.
3. Never go for long periods without food. Consume snacks in a manner which best coincides with the hours when your particular insulin has its maximum effect—two to four hours for the short-acting insulins, six to eight hours for the intermediate insulins, twelve to sixteen hours for the prolonged insulins.
4. Snacks taken between meals or during exercise should be proteins or fats. The effect of carbohydrates in raising the blood sugar is not suffi-

ciently prolonged for an effective preventative. Fats and proteins, on the other hand, prolong the glycemic effect of food over a period of several hours.

5. Always carry with you some type of carbohydrate (sugar, candy, etc.) in case hypoglycemic symptoms occur.

These few rules, once thoroughly understood, can become as much a part of the diabetic's subconscious way of dealing with possible insulin reactions as the rules he or she learned in childhood about preventing colds. If this seems unrealistically positive, consider the case of the elderly lady who, after having taken insulin for many years, was told that her condition had improved to such a point that her insulin could be discontinued.

The woman could not accept this diagnosis, refusing to be deprived of her insulin regimen, and in an attempt to have it reinstated, she insisted on having her blood sugar checked needlessly several times before her next scheduled office visit. In addition, she insisted that eating without insulin might aggravate her diabetes. As a result, she curtailed her diet and lost several pounds, although she had previously been at her proper weight. In short, the woman became so agitated that it was necessary to substitute a small dose of insulin daily as a placebo, after which she reverted to her previous, well-balanced state.

The oral drugs

"Since our daughter doesn't like needles couldn't we substitute one of the oral insulins?"

I'm afraid there are no oral insulins. Insulin can only be administered via injection. The anti-diabetic oral drugs available today work in other ways to reduce high blood glucose.

These drugs cannot help everyone, but for many diabetics they are, as one of my patients put it, "the answer to a prayer." I vividly recall the tremendous wave of enthusiasm that swept through the medical profession some twenty years ago when the early reports on these drugs were presented. At one meeting every seat in the auditorium was occupied and some doctors, their dignified images notwithstanding, were almost literally hanging from the rafters in order to hear the presentation. Their hopes were not exaggerated.

Many diabetics were taken off insulin and switched to oral medication, and many others who could not (or would not) be controlled through dietary measures alone, responded favorably to them. Today, these drugs are used successfully by approximately one-third of all diabetic patients.

There are two basic types of oral drugs:

1. *Sulfonylureas:* These drugs produce a lowering of the blood glucose by stimulating the release of insulin from the patient's own pancreas. It follows that for the drugs to be effective, the patient's pancreas must be able to make and store insulin, and this ability is found chiefly in diabetics who have developed the disease after the age of forty or fifty years. Examples of the sulfonylureas are: Orinase (tolbutamide), Diabinese (chlorpropamide), Dymelor (acetohexamide), and Tolinase (tolazamide).

2. *Biguanides:* It is still not clear how these drugs work—some theories suggest they increase the utilization of blood glucose by muscle and other tissue, and some that they slow down the rate of absorption of carbohydrates from the bowel. None of these theories is entirely sufficient, but

whatever the mechanism, they definitely do
work, and are mainly used for middle-aged and
elderly persons who are not responsive to the
sulfonylureas and for patients for whom the sulfonylureas have been only partially successful.
The chief example of the biguanides is DBI
(phenformin).

I have concerned myself chiefly with drugs and their
use in this chapter, but there are a great many more
questions on the patient's mind: How do I keep control
of my diabetes? What can I eat and drink? What about
my children? How do I avoid complications? What if
my child already has diabetes? What about exercise?
Why do different doctors give me different instructions? All these questions and many others will be
answered in the following chapters. Let's start with
the first one.

3

KEEPING
CONTROL

WHEN A PATIENT'S diabetes has been brought under control, how is the control to be maintained? The answer is an easy-to-follow regimen, carefully tailored to the individual's needs and habits. All too often, however, the diabetic is given a program too complicated or impractical to follow, and nowhere is this more true than in the area of self-testing to keep track of blood and urine glucose levels. Testing is a vital part of the diabetic's program, but he often fails to do the testing exactly as told or, even if he does follow instructions, fails to achieve the desired readings. He disappoints his doctor, his family and, very often, himself. The result: a major cause of diabetic neurosis.

A young housewife, four months pregnant, told me, "I do the best I can with the way I've been told to control my diabetes. I try to stick with my diet and my insulin, and I make my urine tests. But my sugar still goes up and down. And my doctor—I don't know why—he yells at me when my tests show sugar, and he yells at me when they don't. I just can't live with that."

A male patient, whose program called for regulation and control via blood glucose tests taken in his doctor's office, complained, "My doctor does the blood sugars okay, but I don't get the results until two days later.

It's past history by then. But if the test shows high sugar, you ought to hear the third degree I get at home about what I've been eating. I'm made to feel guilty and I don't even know why or what good it's supposed to do."

A different side of the same problem was presented by the wife of a forty-year-old newly diagnosed diabetic. She was very near tears when she came to me. "Our doctor told me how important it is for my husband to make his urine tests. He wants the tests made three times a day and a record kept. But my husband has stopped doing it. Another salesman where he works says the tests aren't accurate, so why bother? So now my husband gets irritated if I keep after him to follow the doctor's orders, but then the doctor criticizes me when my husband doesn't do it. I'm at my wits' end."

The other salesman, it turned out, was also a diabetic and had been told by his doctor that urine tests made by the patient were virtually worthless in the control of diabetes. Which doctor was correct? And why the conflicting advice?

To properly answer these questions, we must look at two different areas of concern:

1. The importance of testing. Is it really necessary?
2. The best method for testing. If testing must be done, who should do it and how?

Importance of testing

Diabetic experts differ on the matter of what level of blood sugar diabetic patients should maintain. The majority opinion, supported by such respected groups as the American Diabetes Association and the Joslin Clinic, holds that the aim should be "normal" blood sugar levels. Other physicians, myself included, are convinced that higher than "normal" sugar levels are of no consequence provided the patient does not demonstrate diabetic symptoms.

Those who support the majority opinion point out that above-normal glucose levels produce sustained stimulation of the pancreas beta cells and, these doctors contend, such over-stimulation will produce exhaustion of the cells. The only support data for this view would appear to be some old, rather questionable animal experiments, however. There is no proof that any organ in the body can be exhausted by transient stimulation.

There is, on the other hand, considerable evidence that the pancreas of some diabetics will respond positively to a high blood sugar level by putting out increased amounts of insulin. In fact, studies in Seattle have shown that when the pancreas is driven by a high carbohydrate diet, glucose tolerance actually improves! And, finally, autopsies of diabetics have tended to show that, despite years of hyperglycemia (too high a blood sugar level), the remaining islets of the pancreas are perfectly normal. What this all means is that higher than usual sugar levels can be all right.

It is also very important to note that striving for "normal" blood glucose levels in the diabetic can be both unrealistic and dangerous. The goals for glucose values generally recommended are these:

Fasting: 60–120 mg. percent
One hour after meals: 200 mg. percent
Two hours after meals: 130 mg. percent
Three hours after meals: 120 mg. percent

While it is true that these goals are realistic for some patients, almost all diabetologists agree that in many cases such levels of control cannot be achieved. The studies of Dr. G. D. Molnar and his colleagues,[1] for example, show that with the treatment now available the diabetic's blood glucose patterns cannot be made to conform to those of normal people.

Every doctor knows full well that diabetes is irreversible; that is, that the distinguishing mark of the disease—elevated blood sugar—cannot be obliterated by any known treatment. Thus, even in their "well-controlled" patients, physicians are *bound* to see moderate elevations of glucose levels that can far exceed the normal levels of a non-diabetic.

The goal of "normalcy" is unrealistic, and efforts to achieve such unrealistic goals soon lead to accusations by the physician as well as by the patient's family that the patient is breaking his regimen. This, in turn, leads to feelings of frustration and guilt on the diabetic's part; and determined to wash away his guilt, he may practice measures so stringent that he errs on the other side, causes his blood sugar to drop too far and develops hypoglycemia.

It is difficult to see how the supposition that an elevation in blood glucose is intrinsically deleterious to the body could be supported. First of all, glucose is a basic constituent of all foods—carbohydrates, proteins, fats. It is also a normal constituent of the blood and essential to the physiologic functions of all the organs in the body—in fact, essential to life itself. The brain, for example, requires glucose for its normal functioning, which explains why hypoglycemia causes loss of consciousness and other serious reactions of the central nervous system.

Moreover, no physician hesitates to administer intravenous glucose, the purest and most concentrated form of sugar there is, to diabetic and non-diabetic alike in the treatment of serious surgical and medical conditions. It is paradoxical that once the intravenous glucose administration is discontinued, the diabetic is again told that he must avoid any food which contains sugar!

In light of the above, it seems senseless to put the

diabetic through a continuous process of testing simply in order to try to correct his blood sugar level to the "normal" glucose levels of the non-diabetic. But where testing *is* important, in fact crucial, is in maintaining control—in making sure that glucose levels remain within proper bounds.

As pointed out in the previous chapter, keeping control is a matter of an ever-changing regimen. Dosage in terms of insulin or oral drugs and, to a lesser extent, diet, should fluctuate constantly, and it is foolhardy to insist on a fixed regimen, especially a fixed insulin dosage.

"But why?" asks the newly diagnosed diabetic. "Once weeks are spent to find the right program for control of my diabetes, why should it have to be changed?"

The answer is simple: The body changes. It changes even if we eat precisely the same foods, perform precisely the same amount of exercise, live in precisely the same environment. Proof of this can be seen in the fact that even under the strictest hospital conditions, patients' blood glucose levels fluctuate markedly. As surely and simply as our appetites vary and our taste preferences change from week to week and month to month, so too do many physical conditions such as the level of glucose in our blood.

The physician cannot be expected to adjust his patient's regimen to glucose changes except through a reliable method of testing, so, yes, testing is necessary, after all. The problem lies with the testing procedures. The ideal program, in order to insure implementation, ought to be almost as simple and mechanical as brushing one's teeth.

Let us consider the testing methods available.

Blood tests

Despite many new refinements in assessing diabetes, blood sugar tests still remain the most acceptable way to identify clinical Diabetes Mellitus. They do present problems, however. First of all, there is the matter of delay in obtaining results.

Hal, a high school math teacher, came to me after a disturbing experience. He had felt badly during one of his classes, left school and gone to his doctor's office for a blood sugar test—only to end up in the hospital before the results of the test were even available.

Why? A blood glucose test can be processed within thirty minutes and even on the most modest schedule two hours should be adequate for any laboratory. The greatest delays often occur in transmitting the results to the patient.

"It's a conspiracy of silence that says only the doctor can discuss such matters with you," insists the mother of a teenage diabetic. "So when you ask the nurse or lab or anybody but the doctor, you are told, 'Your physician will tell you,' and he usually does, but after how long?"

Patients and their families also complain about the confusion surrounding the mechanics of the blood test. In most cases today, the blood is tested two hours *after* the meal, but not long ago diabetics were forbidden to eat before a blood test. Some labs test whole blood, while others test plasma, and the levels that result are quite different, plasma readings being in general some fifteen percent higher than whole blood determinations.

In addition, interference in the measurement of blood glucose may be caused by drugs and by constituents of blood and urine which react in the same way as glucose. In the presence of vitamin C, for example, glucose may be underestimated, while the exact opposite is true in the presence of tetracyclines. Ingestion of large amounts of fruit may also give rise to falsely raised glucose values. In all of these cases, the false answers are not easy to detect in a single blood glucose test because of the wide range of possible values. Many of the current methods for testing blood glucose yield values which can be considered as suspect.

At best, the results of an isolated blood glucose test reflect only momentary information—the sugar level at a single point in time. The blood glucose may undergo considerable change in a few minutes before or after the sample is taken: an elevated blood sugar can drop to hypoglycemic levels in only two hours. To be meaningful, therefore, several blood tests must be conducted in a twenty-four-hour period. And here we encounter the most serious limitation of blood sugar tests: they must be carried out in the doctor's office or a hospital.

If a convenient method were available to measure the blood glucose level throughout the twenty-four-hour day, this, in spite of all the other shortcomings, would still be the method of choice for evaluating diabetic control. To date, however, there is only one procedure available for use by diabetics themselves and it cannot be recommended; first, because the accuracy is highly suspect, and second, because the procedure requires a finger prick with a needle several times a day and, therefore, is not likely to be carried out regularly enough by the patient.

Hospitals

Since multiple readings in a twenty-four-hour period are essential if blood sugar tests are to be meaningful, some physicians recommend periodic hospitalization as a method for monitoring the status of the disease. Although this procedure may solve the problem of convenience, I cannot recommend it due to a host of other problems it produces.

Patients complain that the care given to hospitalized diabetics is generally dreadful, and the staff has little or no idea of the diabetic's special requirements. "You may get your insulin early and then be forced to wait two hours for breakfast," one patient complained. "And try to get a glass of orange juice out of someone in a hospital. It's impossible."

Getting a snack of any kind can also prove difficult. The doctor of one patient brought in sugar cubes in case of an insulin reaction, and a nurse saw the cubes and actually took them away, in spite of the patient's protests, insisting that the cubes must be there for "cheating." Not surprisingly, many patients come to believe that nurses simply do not know enough about diabetes, and that physicians do not realize how pervasive this ignorance is.

In some hospitals, nurses are even given the responsibility for prescribing insulin dosage, often with disastrous results. As one patient described the situation, "They took blood sugars regularly, and when my sugar was high, the nurse would add insulin. Later in the evening, I went into insulin shock." In my experience, the treating physician must be on guard constantly to protect the diabetic patient from carelessness and ignorance on the part of hospital personnel, often including supposedly well-trained house officers.

Most important of all, however, is the fact that the in-hospital insulin dosage for the patient rarely proves to be satisfactory when he or she goes home. The environment (absence of family and friends, etc.), the quality of exercise and the meals, all tend to be quite different in the hospital as compared to home. In addition, the telescoping of insulin increments—from three or four shots of regular insulin in the hospital to one or two shots of regular and long-acting insulin at home—frequently leads to hypoglycemia and the need to back-pedal the insulin dosage at home This reduction, in turn, tends to produce excessive hyperglycemia, and the patient may soon find his diabetes totally out of control.

It follows that hospitalization very often invites more harm than help.

Urine testing

In view of these limitations on blood testing, it is necessary to use another method for gauging the level of glucose in the blood: urine testing. It has been found that when the blood glucose level exceeds a certain threshold (about 150 to 200 mg. percent), it then begins to appear in the urine and, thus, the quantity of sugar in the urine of a diabetic patient closely reflects the blood sugar level.

Unlike sugar tests of the blood, urine tests may be made by the patient without fear of pain (no needle pricks) and with a greater degree of regularity. Even so, I strongly recommend that urine testing conducted to maintain diabetic control be carried out by the physician rather than the patient. Let me explain why:

First, although self-testing urine methods are more reliable than self-testing methods for blood sugar, the urine methods are far from foolproof. Jerome Feldman and Francine Lebovitz[2] point out that errors can occur with a number of brand names. In a study on the misleading results of tests for glycosuria, they report that one brand of tablets gave falsely high sugar tests in 111 of 172 specimens—sixty-five percent!

As Clifford Gastineau points out,[8] error can also arise because the various methods of testing urine (stick, tape and tablet) use different percentages for the different marks on the scale (Negative, Grade 1,

Grade 2, Grade 3 and Grade 4). Moreover, these tests are not as accurate as the percentage marks on the scale might lead one to believe. The marks indicate only approximate values, and none of these tests are reliable when the concentration of glucose exceeds one-half percent.

Again, various medications such as vitamin C can affect the reaction in the test paper so as to distort the results of a test. Improper washing of the test tube and eyedropper can be another common source of error—a false positive test can result from contamination by a four-plus urine left over from a previous test —and the most significant misleading factor of all seems to be the urine *volume*. If the individual has drunk a large amount of water, the same amount of sugar will have a lower concentration than in a lesser volume of urine.

From all of this, the conclusion is inescapable that there is an exceedingly great potential for misleading tests among most diabetic patients who perform self-testing—and that if the results of these are relied upon to evaluate diabetes control, then many errors in treatment are possible.

Dr. John Burrington, professor of surgery and pediatrics at the University of Chicago Pritzker School of Medicine, points out another hazard. He reported to the annual meeting of the Society of Thoracic Surgeons at Montreal[4] on five children between the ages of nineteen and twenty-six months who incurred full-thickness burns of the esophagus after swallowing a particular indicator tablet. All developed such severe narrowing of the passage that they were untreatable by repeated dilation, and surgery was eventually required.

When a tablet is swallowed by a child, he reported, it apparently dissolved in saliva to form a sludge that sticks in the esophagus about the level of the carina and causes a severe burn, both by its caustic nature and by the large local release of heat. Narrowing of the passages then develops over the following three to four months. The acute symptoms are often surprisingly mild so that the child may not be brought to the physician's attention until the developing stricture interferes with swallowing.

Dr. Burrington said that both patients and their physicians are insufficiently acquainted with the hazards of these tablets. In one case, the child's father actually saw him swallow the tablet but was unaware of the danger and so did not seek medical help until the next day when the child was feverish, breathing irregularly and unable to swallow his saliva.

In another case, a child was brought to the hospital after he had experienced difficulty in swallowing for a two-week period. Although persistent questioning of the child eventually enabled the physician to relate the symptoms to the pill, neither he nor the parents had been aware of the tablet's caustic nature. Dr. Burrington also points out that this is something to be aware of even if there is no diabetes in the child's immediate family—two of the five children he treated had swallowed the offending tablets while visiting in another home.

Dr. Burrington noted that vinegar and lemon juice are listed as antidotes on the bottle, but expressed the belief that they may do more harm than good. While it seems logical to neutralize the caustic base with these acids, he said, the neutralization reaction intensified the release of heat, and the preferred antidote is cold milk, which also has the advantage of being readily available and acceptable to the child.

Although danger to children and lack of accuracy are major drawbacks to the use of urine self-testing for diabetics, far more important is the mental anguish such testing can produce. The layman, however intelligent and cooperative, is simply not sufficiently trained to interpret test results properly. Consider these fairly typical cases:

E.W., a thirty-four-year-old plumber, told me this story on his first visit to my office: "My diabetes has been very unpredictable, with wild swings from heavy sugar to insulin reactions. Not long ago, while I had a sore throat, very heavy sugar began to appear in my urine. Despite the fact that I ate very little, the tests continued to show sugar. Finally, I had to go to the hospital. I was very ill and had to be given large amounts of insulin and fluid in the vein. I don't want that to happen again."

E.W.'s "wild swings" were at the root of his trouble, and these grew directly out of the fact that he had been instructed to test his own urine. Upon consistently finding two-plus and three-plus tests, he became emotionally upset, berated himself for eating the wrong foods and began restricting his diet so severely that he soon suffered hypoglycemia—in other words, he went from one extreme to the other.

On his first visit to my office, I instructed him to eat an afternoon snack (e.g. a small dish of ice cream) each day to avert insulin reactions. On the first day of taking the snack, however, the patient (continuing his self-testing against my recommendation) became so perturbed by a positive urine test that he discontinued the snack and again experienced an insulin reaction, the very thing which had so disturbed him in the first place.

An elderly patient of mine with well-controlled diabetes took a Florida vacation with her husband to visit her sister. The latter, accustomed to testing her husband's urine, offered to test my patient's as well. Upon doing so, she exclaimed, "Your sugar is bad!" That was all my patient needed to hear. She promptly felt "weak and sick all over." The results of this single urine test frightened her so much that she aborted her vacation and returned home a week earlier than she had planned.

Her family physician, whom she consulted for her

sudden sickness, listened to the story of what had happened and then shunted her off by stating, "Your symptoms are due to your sugar." Concluding from this statement that her diabetes was out of control, she restricted her diet severely; this, in turn, produced a weight loss, which the patient wrongly attributed to the excess sugar her sister had reported originally.

When finally she came to me, my tests revealed that her diabetes was perfectly controlled, as had always been the case in previous examinations. The symptoms which she had developed were all of mental origin, triggered by a urine test performed by a layman who lacked sufficient knowledge to properly interpret information.

A twenty-three-year-old female developed the classic symptoms of diabetes one year before consulting me. She felt very well after the diabetes was regulated with insulin, but she was also conducting urine tests four times daily. She read in a diabetic manual that her urine must be negative at all times, and as a result she became frustrated and anxious when the tests revealed even a small amount of sugar—despite her doctor's statement that such fluctuations were to be expected.

Many doctors instruct their patients to "test yourself in the morning before breakfast and again at noon before lunch." As a result, patients assume the doctor is concerned about insulin reaction, so the patient becomes fearful when the urine test is negative for sugar. Other patients take extra insulin when the urine test is four-plus, and they take orange juice if it is negative. Worse yet, the concept of "good" and "bad" urine tests implies almost a behavioral judgment that may provoke unnecessary anxiety for the patient who has "bad" tests.

Diabetic authorities such as the Joslin Clinic have devised formulas to guide patients in adjusting their insulin dosage according to the results of urine tests

—insulin to be increased five units for one-plus, ten units for two-plus, fifteen units for three-plus and twenty units for four-plus. As a result, it has become customary for doctors to advise diabetic patients to follow this procedure. Some physicians even provide every newly diagnosed diabetic with a notebook to keep careful account of his urine tests, and instruct him to bring it in on each visit so that the physician may evaluate his daily progress. The doctor may insert a written comment to further emphasize his concern about day-to-day progress.

From all this, it is only natural for a patient to conclude that the urine should be sugar-free twenty-four hours per day, a goal which is both unrealistic and dangerous. While such a goal may seem to work for a time, it is based on false premises. States Dr. Gastineau: "The body must have a certain amount of carbohydrate and enough insulin to use it. If it does not have both, the body starts to burn fat and protein at an excessive rate, and ketone bodies are formed. Decreasing the amount of food eaten in order to correct an excessive amount of sugar in the urine is poor practice, because it tends to increase the production of ketones and leads to confusion in knowing the amount of insulin needed."[5]

Equally important, the doctor goes on to say, "No major harm seems to be done by brief periods of excess sugar. In summary, it is best to adhere to your usual diet plan at all times, even if the urine tests show sugar."

Some doctors advocate alterations in insulin dosage by the patient to match changes in sugar levels, but I cannot subscribe to this practice. It fails to take into account the fluctuations of blood and urine sugar which occur in diabetics not only from day to day but even from hour to hour, as documented by Molnar and his colleagues.[6] Any attempt to correct these fluctuations by altering the insulin dose after the fact can be hazardous. A patient's blood sugar may drop precipitously following an injection of extra insulin and, as happens all too frequently in such situations, cause an insulin reaction. Those who advise such frequent alterations fail to take into consideration one important fact: there is a lag of at least forty-eight hours before a change of insulin dosage has any kind of noticeable effect. Molnar found that an increase of the insulin doses designed to bring the blood sugar to normal not only failed to reduce the blood sugar but increased the frequency and severity of hypoglycemic episodes, due to this factor.

The essence of Molnar's studies is very simple: variations in the blood sugar occur despite keeping insulin, diet and exercise constant from day to day —yet these are the very elements blamed by the diabetic and his physician for fluctuations in sugar content. If the patient then increases the insulin dosage, based on self-testing, it only serves to aggravate the situation—more insulin reactions followed by more sugar in the urine—and the patient and his family become demoralized. The patient tends to assume responsibility for the failure, and this leads to frustration, guilt, anxiety and a very unhappy day-to-day existence.

Dr. Harrison Sadler, at a postgraduate course sponsored by the American Diabetes Association, reported that psychiatric evaluations of twenty-five recent adult-onset diabetics revealed that seven were depressed and fourteen emotionally disturbed.[7] Sadler recognized, as do all physicians who treat diabetes, that the diabetic patient is no longer self-reliant when he says things like "To hell with it," or "Why should this happen after all I've done?" Such a patient becomes forgetful, provocative and manipulative in what can be called the "masochistic" stage of the disease.

In his brief encounter with diabetics (and with only a small sample at that), Dr. Sadler very perceptively recognized the predominance of psychiatric abnormalities. His suggested "cure," on the other hand, was not so perceptive. To help such depressed patients, Dr. Sadler recommended increased participation in their own sugar monitoring and in their regimen adjustments. Unwittingly, he had recommended a cure that was one of the chief causes of the problem. I cannot agree that the way to improve the mental state of diabetics who are depressed or have "given up" is to make them become their own physician and, thereby, hold them to account for any fluctuations in glucose levels. It would only depress them further, and unfairly so.

In my judgment, the only answer to such emotional disturbances is to remove the responsibility for his disease from the diabetic patient's shoulders and put it on the more stable ones of a physician who is confident and skilled in the management of diabetes. This relief permits the patient to carry out other, more rewarding activities of daily living, such as school and work.

True, it frequently happens that physicians themselves become upset upon finding an elevated blood sugar when they test their patient's urine, but with their medical background and experience in handling other diabetic patients, they are far better prepared to cope with the situation. The self-testing diabetic patient, on the other hand, has no such background or experience—yet urine testing places him in a position of evaluating and interpreting a test for which he is totally unprepared. End result: diabetic neurosis.

Recommended procedure

Once a patient's diabetes is well-controlled, the basic objective for any testing program is to maintain that control, and this can best be accomplished by a program which:

1. Is extremely reliable.
2. Is simple for the patient to implement.
3. Helps to ease the patient's concerns rather than causing or aggravating them.

The method which best answers these requirements is monthly testing by the physician of twenty-four-hour fractional urines. Let me explain this procedure.

The patient selects a day—perhaps the first Saturday or Sunday of every month—and during this full twenty-four-hour period keeps a record of the total amount of urine passed for the following day segments:

1. After breakfast to before lunch.
2. After lunch to before dinner.
3. After dinner to before bed.
4. After rising to before breakfast.

The patient saves the urine during each of these periods, records the volume and keeps a one-ounce portion before flushing the rest away.

For example, the patient saves in a large container all the urine passed from right after breakfast until lunchtime. The amount of urine in this container is recorded and a sample placed in a vial supplied by the physician, then the remainder flushed away and the large container cleaned. Then the patient repeats the procedure from lunch until dinner. In this way, he is able to take to his physician four separate urine samples, each clearly labeled to indicate a) which of the four periods it is from, and b) the total volume of urine collected for that period.

In the physician's office or laboratory, each of the urine samples is carefully tested for the percentage of sugar, then this percentage is multiplied by the urine volume. In this way, the physician can determine the exact amount of glucose for each of the four periods. If, for example, there is a low morning count and a high evening reading, additional long-acting insulin might be indicated, while a high morning reading and a low evening count might indicate the need for additional regular insulin.

The quantitative nature of this test is extremely important and can be readily understood by considering the following example. Suppose a lunch-to-dinner urine sample showed a sugar percentage of 1.0 percent. If the quantity of urine for this period were eight ounces (240cc), the grams of sugar lost for this period would be 2.4, an amount within reasonable limits. But if the urine volume were sixteen ounces (480cc), then the sugar lost would be 4.8 grams, a loss which has passed the bounds of good control.

There are several ways in which your physician may test the fractional urine samples, but I strongly recommend the Somogyi method. I have found it to be eminently satisfactory, both in accuracy and simplicity.

The test is performed by carmelizing the urinary sugar with a ten percent sodium carbonate solution. In a process similar to making candy on top of the stove, five ml. of sodium carbonate is boiled in a water bath for eight minutes along with 0.5 ml. of the patient's urine. The physician then compares the color of the carmelized product with the colors on the Somogyi colorimeter (varying shades of brown with values ranging from 0.5 percent to 6 percent) to determine the percentage of sugar in the patient's urine sample. This percentage multiplied by the urine volume gives the exact amount of glucose in grams.

This procedure cannot be carried out with the necessary precision by the patient at home. It must be done in the doctor's office or laboratory, not only because when the patient brings twenty-four-hour specimens to the physician for analysis and recommendations, he can be assured of accuracy in the testing—but because the patient is also completely relieved of the responsibility for evaluating his or her own diabetes control, a responsibility which is one of the chief causes of diabetic neurosis.

The relief from performing daily urine tests has an extremely positive effect on the emotional state of the diabetic. It is, in fact, an effect which often defies description. Ernie, a professional golf instructor, illustrates the point:

"How could I teach golf when I couldn't get my head together? Now it's totally different since I quit doing the testing. The other doctors were always after me with 'How has your sugar been? Are you testing every day?' And what really used to drive me up the wall was that I would find sugar in my urine at a time when I felt like I was on the verge of a hypoglycemic effect!"

Perhaps Ernie's wife summed it up best of all when she told me, "Since you took over the responsibility for his diabetes, Ernie isn't worried anymore."

4

FOOD AND DRINK

THE ENTIRE SUBJECT of food and drink for the diabetic is filled with problems defined by the American Medical Association as "nutritional neurosis and food faddism." No other aspect of life causes the diabetic and his family so much anxiety, guilt and confusion.

"My cousin is a physician's assistant," a new patient, a very attractive woman in her mid-thirties, told me, "so the minute I said they'd found sugar in my urine, my cousin said it was good-bye to happy eating. No more cake or pie or anything like that. Just the thought of it depressed me terribly."

"My wife told me I'd have to quit sweets cold," said another patient, a large man with a very hardy appetite. "I haven't had a decent meal since."

Imagine the psychological consequences of such advice in today's world, bombarded as we are by constant invitations to eat, drink and consume—on television, in newspapers and magazines, in the grocery store. Aside from any pangs of personal deprivation, consider what it means in terms of family togetherness for the diabetic mother who draws "great pleasure from preparing special desserts for my family," or for the diabetic father who has always enjoyed "going out for an ice cream" with his family.

"I know I shouldn't eat some of the things I do," says E.R., "but there are lots of subtle pressures most people never even think about." So E.R., like most diabetics, goes on eating so-called "forbidden" foods and suffering doubly, first, because of his efforts to restrain himself, and second, because of his guilty conscience each time he fails.

"My son is a teenager," the mother of a diabetic told me. "I can't get him to stick with his diet. It's so confusing, he says he can't even understand it, much less follow it, and I have to agree with him. But it scares me."

Over the years, a special language has grown up around dieting for diabetics. Terms such as "free diets," "strict diets" and "diabetic diets" abound, causing misinterpretation by patients, clinicians and physicians alike and leading to either anger or apathy on the part of many diabetics when they can't follow them as "strictly" as they think they should. "I can't take those diabetic diets," new patients often tell me. "They're not fair to me or to my family. They're so structured they're oppressive. No sweets, all that measuring. It's like having a keeper."

Such diets, which demand that patients alter not only their natural taste preferences but even their life-styles, are doomed to failure. It is not surprising that fifty to eighty percent of diabetics fail to follow the dietary advice they are given.

These restrictions and prohibitions are equally difficult for the family of the diabetic. They deny themselves "sweet stuff" for fear of putting temptation in harm's way or, just as psychologically dangerous, feel guilty each time they do succumb. "I know it's not fair to the rest of the family," says the mother of an eleven-year-old diabetic daughter, "but if I served any sweet things at the table, it would make me feel terrible for my little girl."

Such problems are not limited to food. "If I have a drink at home," says the wife of a diabetic, "I try to hide what I'm doing. That makes me feel like an alcoholic, but if I don't hide it, I wonder if my husband is looking at me and feeling deprived."

Meanwhile, that woman's husband, the former president of a social club, refuses to go out with his old group of friends. "If I can't take a drink," he explains, "I'll put a damper on everybody else's time."

So patients and their families suffer from fear of drinking, embarrassment at not drinking, fear of overeating, fear of undereating, guilt due to "going off my diet," difficulties in staying on—and absolutely none of this is necessary.

The truth is that diabetics, with good counseling, a proper understanding of their condition and a reasonable amount of will power, can eat and drink in a manner sufficient not only to satisfy their own inner needs, but to make their families tend to forget their diabetes—and to keep friends and acquaintances totally unaware of it.

The medical evidence is clear: neither sweets nor alcohol are, in themselves, harmful to diabetics. Since the forceable removal of these items from the diet can produce severe neurosis in diabetics and their families, this alone is ample reason to make certain that the age-old stigma against such items is erased. But there is more. The evidence is also clear that the removal of such sources of carbohydrate from the diabetic's diet can do physical as well as psychological harm. It can result in dangerously lowered levels of energy on the one hand, and increased levels of cholesterol and triglyceride (cholesterol-related fatty acid) on the other.

In view of such evidence, why do so many "authorities" appear to believe otherwise? What is the reason for the layers upon layers of misinformation? Why isn't the truth not common knowledge?

The answer lies in the nature and history of diabetes.

Nature and history

Derived from Greek words meaning "passing through honey," the name Diabetes Mellitus refers to the elevated glucose (blood sugar) in a patient's urine. The patient's glucose surplus passes from the bloodstream through the kidneys into the urine, causing the disease's characteristic symptoms: extreme thirst, hunger, weakness, weight loss and abnormally large amounts of urine.

Let's go back to the last century and try to visualize what a physician thought when faced with the challenge of fighting such a disease. With only a minimal knowledge of the subject and no blood tests or urinalysis to verify clinical findings, his diagnostic technique was limited almost entirely to the study of patient symptoms. Noting the patient's frequent urination, then, he would logically have taken a urine specimen and compared it with one from a normal individual. Perhaps he noted the number of flies attracted to the diabetic urine, perhaps he actually tasted the specimens, for whatever reason, he became aware of the high sugar content.

The conclusion was natural: the source of this excess sugar was the high-sugar foods consumed by the patient, and so he advised his patient to deny himself all sweets. Could that physician have been expected to know that the patient's excess blood sugar was due to the *shortage* of a commodity (insulin), not to the overabundance of one?

"Sweets are poison to the diabetic," says an ancient medical text. Thus were the seeds of diabetic diet neurosis sown—and their growth would be stimulated by every major medical advance in the field of diabetics.

In 1916, five years before the discovery of insulin,

Frederick M. Allen took several dogs and removed seven-eighths of the pancreas from each. The result: on a normal diet, the dogs died in a diabetic coma—but even with that one-eighth of a pancreas they were able to survive and live a normal life span *if they were fed a low-calorie diet.* This startling principle was then applied with great success to human diabetics.

There are two types of diabetics: the juvenile diabetic, whose pancreas fails to produce any insulin at all; and the adult-onset diabetic (by far the greatest number) whose pancreas produces some insulin but not enough. Dr. Allen's low-calorie diet could not save the lives of juvenile or thin or normal-weight insulin-deficient diabetics, but for obese individuals whose problem was an overburdened pancreas producing reduced amounts of insulin, it brought impressive results. In most instances, diabetes control was achieved rapidly, and occasionally the condition even reverted to normal.

The benefits of this diet regimen, as Dr. Allen sought to emphasize throughout his studies, were a result of the low-calorie content and its effect on the overweight condition of the patients. Their diabetic condition improved because they limited the number of calories they consumed, not because there was a limit on the *kinds* of food they could enjoy.

In spite of Dr. Allen's efforts to place emphasis where it belonged, however, his discovery was constantly linked to the ancient theory that sugar in the urine meant sugar in the diet. Because a reduction in carbohydrate almost invariably means a reduction in calories, most medical authorities in America decided that Dr. Allen's experiments had been successful not because they offered a diet low in calories, but because they offered one low in sweets.

Even the great discovery of insulin in 1921 by Banting and Best did not begin to set the record straight. With the lives of insulin-deficient adult and juvenile diabetics now preserved and their primary defect counteracted by way of insulin injections, one would expect that the next logical step in the treatment of diabetes would have been the reassessment and normalization of food and drink consumption.

But no, the ingrown custom of restricting carbohydrates in diabetic patients persisted—so much so that diabetic children, although their insulin deficiency had now been corrected, frequently lacked sufficient energy to attend classes because of low-carbohydrate diets! Worse yet, many of these children, failing to attain normal growth and development, became "diabetic dwarfs."

"Sweets are poison to the diabetic," said the history books, and in spite of new discoveries, the authorities refused to believe otherwise.

Not until 1930, almost ten years after the discovery of insulin, was a beginning made in the prescription of larger quantities of carbohydrates for diabetic patients. Dr. Sansum in Santa Barbara, California, pioneered it, but the advantages of his diets over the usual noncarbohydrate ones were "discovered" in a most unusual fashion.

It was not uncommon for diabetics who vacationed in California and were cared for by Dr. Sansum to report to their doctors in New York that they felt much better while vacationing in Santa Barbara, only to revert to feeling fatigued and lethargic after returning home. At first, the New York doctors were inclined to attribute the improved health to the California climate, but ultimately it became clear that the beneficial effects resulted from the additional carbohydrates permitted in Dr. Sansum's diets.

The message was plain: increasing sweets, as long as calories were kept sufficiently low in other ways, not only provided psychological benefits, but also reduced lethargy. It was a message soon to be supported by the 1935 high-carbohydrate, low-calorie diet experiments of Dr. Himsworth in England—yet it never filtered down to the diabetic and his family. Most medical authorities continued to preach the same old sermon: "Sweets are poison to the diabetic."

"If Western clinicians had been less parochial, we would have appreciated sooner the surprising tolerance of diabetics for dietary carbohydrate when caloric intake is controlled."[1] So says Dr. K. M. West, who reported in 1973 that many Eastern and tropical nations had long known that diabetics could be satisfactorily controlled by diets containing almost twice as much carbohydrate as that in the diabetic diets of the West.

The diabetics in one Japanese clinic, for example, consumed sixty-four percent of their calories in carbohydrates, and in India, clinicians often prescribed diets that contained more than seventy percent carbohydrate content. It is worth noting here that a meal of the typical, nondiabetic Asian is low in calories and, in terms of percentage, high in carbohydrates, some one hundred thirty to two hundred fifty grams—and that Asians have a very low incidence of diabetes.

Today, evidence of both the physical and psychological benefits of high-carbohydrate, low-calorie diets for diabetics continues to grow. Consider these more recent examples:

- The diabetic patients of Stone and Conner did well on diets containing sixty-five percent of the calories as carbohydrates.[2]
- In 1949, Dr. K. M. West, treating a severe diabetic with malignant hypertension, "out of desperation" prescribed a rice diet. Although this increased the patient's dietary carbohydrate by almost three hundred percent, no increase in insulin was necessary.
- Later, Dr. West studied a severe diabetes patient on a standard diabetic diet. After a suitable

control period in a metabolic ward, the patient's daily carbohydrate consumption was doubled (from one hundred eighty to three hundred sixty grams), which greatly improved the patient's energy level and general sense of wellbeing yet made no change in the levels of blood and urine glucose.

- R. L. Weinsier showed that for eighteen diabetic patients a diet high in carbohydrate (sixty percent) did not upset the control of diabetes.[3]
- Perhaps the most impressive studies to date are those by J. D. Brunzell and associates. In these experiments, diabetes subjects treated with insulin or oral sulfonylureas all had *lower* fasting glucose levels while receiving the high-carbohydrate diet than they did when receiving the usual diabetic diet.[4]
- Additional studies have also shown that the high-carbohydrate diets, which are low in fat, decrease cholesterol and triglyceride levels.

However, even though these medical studies provide conclusive proof that a low-carbohydrate diet is not indicated in the treatment of diabetes, that, in fact, such a diet can be both physically and psychologically injurious, the notion that "sweets are poison" *still* continues to dominate the thinking of physicians treating diabetes. Why? Because:

1. Old superstitions die hard.
2. Many physicians see that a restriction of carbohydrate intake results in improvement in the diabetic—but fail to recognize that this is actually a result of decreased calories rather than decreased sweets.
3. It seems common sense to connect sugar in the blood with sugar in the mouth. The correlation between the two appears as irrefutable as the

logic which caused a small boy to believe he had caused the East Coast blackout because all the lights went out just as he struck a light pole with his stick.

For these reasons, the false connection between carbohydrates and diabetes, although disproven time and time again, continues to reappear in textbooks and clinics. To this day, the limiting of dietary carbohydrates is the cornerstone of diabetic therapy for most clinicians, dieticians and physicians.

This is not the only restriction to pose mental and physical problems for the diabetic and his family, however. There is also the diet regimen itself.

The diets

Diets prescribed for diabetes not only restrict carbohydrates, they also require very precise measurement of food intake, complex food exchanges and meticulous calorie counting. Since the physician usually emphasizes diet as the keystone of diabetic management, patients and their families naturally jump to the conclusion that whenever they have fluctuations in their glucose readings, errors in calculating food intake, whether accidental or purposeful, are the principal causes.

In truth, however, the human body is a very complex machine, which reacts to a vast array of stimuli. Any attempt to tie changes in blood sugar levels to fluctuations in food consumption would be as foolish as insisting that we get depressed because we eat corned beef and cabbage.

Contrary to the belief of many, the diabetic patient is not likely to gorge himself with food one day and starve the next, any more than any other member of the public. No matter what food idiosyncrasies an individual has, one fact stands out: his menu contains almost identical food items day after day, meal after meal, sometimes to the point of monotony. Most people eat unvarying breakfasts and lunches throughout their lives. Diabetics are as conformist in their eating pattern as anyone else, and the fluctuations in their blood sugar levels and urine sugar tests cannot be correlated with hypothetical peaks and valleys in their food intake. When sugar appears in the urine or the blood sugar is unduly elevated, the patient is utterly blameless.

Even in a hospital there are marked fluctuations in a patient's test results, yet this is one of the most controlled environments a diabetic patient can encounter: all the food is carefully measured and supervised by a dietician, and even the amount of the patient's physical activity is constant. Certainly the patient should not be held responsible for variations of blood and urine sugar under such controlled conditions, yet variations very definitely do occur. How can the patient be blamed?

There are other major areas of confusion. Not too long ago more than two hundred and fifty different diets were being prescribed for diabetics at Cleveland, Ohio's, Mount Sinai Hospital alone! Most of these diets varied from one another by only a few grams of carbohydrate, protein or fat—according to the whim of the physician. Imagine the confusion and uncertainty this caused among diabetics and their families as they compared notes. Even today, although the American Diabetes Association has attempted to reduce the number of diets, the lack of agreement among experts over this subject, as well as over many other aspects of dieting, fosters continued uncertainty.

The complexity and confusion of the diets are not the only self-defeating factors. Quite often the diets call for types of food or preparation so different from the family routine that they become disruptive. The inclusion of expensive "diabetic foods" can become a financial burden. And, most important, too often doctors and dieticians fail to tailor a diet to fit the bodily requirements and life style of the patient. Men who require twenty-five hundred or even thirty-five hundred calories per day, for example, are given diets containing only eighteen hundred calories. Such errors are made for thin men as well as for heavy, women as well as children. Why?

First, many physicians fail to take into account the relationship between calorie requirements and such factors as body size and normal daily exercise.

Second, doctors and dieticians, as well as patients themselves, can overlook the special caloric needs of underweight diabetics.

Third, and of striking importance, many patients are sent home from the hospital on a prescription, such as an eighteen-hundred-calorie ADA diet, which satisfied them perfectly while they were inactive in the hospital, but which will be dangerously deficient for daily activities at home.

Fourth, the increased bulk of the diabetic diet may actually offer a volume of food equal to that to which the patient had been accustomed on a normal diet. For this reason, most diabetics are *initially* satisfied with diets offering only seventy to eighty percent of their actual caloric requirement. But the key word here is "initially." Dissatisfaction soon sets in as the patient is faced with mounting hunger and fatigue.

Small wonder that although all diabetics may claim to be "on a diet," a giant percentage of them do not follow their prescribed diets. The statistical evidence is clear:

- A National Health Survey in Holland showed that twenty-five percent of the diabetics, although admitting they had received a diet, did not follow it, while another twenty-two percent insisted they had never been given a diet at all.[5]
- Among a representative group of American dia-

betics, forty-seven percent failed to follow a prescribed diet.

- Dr. Harvey Knowles and his colleagues summarized seven studies of juvenile diabetics which showed that twenty-two to eighty-nine percent failed to follow their diets.[6]

- In one of the more recent British studies (Tunbridge), seventy percent of the diabetics failed to consume within ten percent of the prescribed amounts of food.

- Studies of the University Group Diabetes Program showed that although significant weight reduction was achieved among all subgroups during the first few days and weeks, old habits soon took over and, as the months passed, adiposity returned.

In many ways, the best of the so-called diabetes diets is the Exchange Diet, developed conjointly by the American Diabetes Association, the American Diabetic Association and the United States Public Health Service. It contains all the essential food ingredients—carbohydrates as well as proteins, fats, fruits, vegetables and milk. The name "Exchange Diet" means that it offers a long list of food items which, based on their calorie count and content of protein, carbohydrate and fat, are interchangeable, thus providing considerable variety.

Even with this diet, however, the complications are such that patients often find it oppressive. Many hours are consumed, for example, in attempting to teach patients the mechanics of the exchange system, and the authors of the diet, although including ice cream and sponge cake in the list of permissible carbohydrates, fall prey to the old "sweets are poison" superstition and advise omission of a long list of "concentrated sugars," such as candy, molasses, honey, jam, jelly, marmalade, syrup, pie, cake, cookies, pastries, condensed milk, soft drinks and candy-coated gum—none of which need be restricted if their caloric value is taken into account.

Thus, in addition to producing and aggravating the emotional traumas I have termed diabetic neurosis, this and other ADA diets may actually be increasing mortality through increased fat consumption. Only recently has the American Diabetes Association, having "discovered" that carbohydrate in the diet has no relationship to diabetic control, promised to liberalize its diets. And in 1971, its expert Committee on Nutrition, taking note of some of the studies cited in this chapter and the potentially deleterious effects of saturated fat, recommended the inclusion of more generous amounts of carbohydrates in such diets.

Unfortunately, however, history has shown that it is extremely difficult for physicians and dieticians to give up the notion that carbohydrates are bad for people with too much sugar in their blood—and the diabetic and his family are in need of help today, not tomorrow.

The following is what I believe to be the best step-by-step approach to the subject of food and drink.

The best approach

PATIENT'S WEIGHT
Before a diet can be prescribed, it is essential to know whether the patient is underweight, overweight or normal. How is this determination to be made?

It is unwise to use the familiar insurance tables for height and weight, since the medical profession has determined these tables to be inaccurate. Insurance companies developed these tables simply by tabulating the weights of their applicants and then drawing an average, and since a cross-section of the American population is overweight, the tables were bound to reflect this obesity.

If one must use such a table, then the "Ideal Weight" is the most satisfactory choice. These weights represent a group of insured who "outlived" their life expectancies (further indication that obesity reduces one's life).

A better and simpler method, however, is observation and judgment by the diabetic and his family. Surprisingly, any group of lay persons will concur as to whether a given individual is underweight, overweight or normal. I have found a very substantial unanimity, for example, among nurses or medical students as to what a patient's weight should be.

At first glance, this method may appear to be too imprecise and unscientific; however, there is one factor that makes it highly recommended: it works.

IF THE PATIENT IS UNDERWEIGHT
The underweight diabetic, like any other undernourished person, not only requires sufficient food for daily physical activities, but additional calories for gaining weight and strength.

Often, the underweight diabetic will regain his weight without an increase in calories due to his diabetes being brought under control by the administration of insulin or oral medication. If this is not the case, however, I prefer to augment the current diet (providing it is nutritionally sound) by additional calories rather than substitute a totally new diet. At first, I simply increase food portions at mealtime and between meals, and if this is not sufficiently productive, I increase the fat content of the diet.

Once the patient has reached normal weight, he should follow the advice given below for those without weight problems.

IF THE PATIENT IS OVERWEIGHT

This includes the vast majority of diabetics. Weight reduction is the prime treatment for their diabetes, and they must adhere strictly to a low-calorie diet, but *only* until they have achieved their normal weight. The low-calorie diet should be just as well balanced nutritionally as any diet, diabetic or not, and it is important to remember that any diet of less than eight hundred calories is unlikely to be able to provide enough essential nutrients to maintain the body over a long period of time without destroying important muscle and other tissue.

I have employed an unlimited meat diet with very good success for many years. By consuming lean meat, fish, chicken and skim milk, a patient will automatically get sufficient protein while at the same time restricting animal fat and cholesterol in his system (see the diet on page 73). Such a diet, while providing all the normal food constituents, also helps the patient establish proper eating habits after he has attained normal weight and is able to follow a maintenance diet.

For the overweight diabetic who regularly follows such a diet, the results are frequently dramatic—in many instances going so far as to reverse the entire diabetic process for an indefinite period. To all intents and purposes, the patient functions as a normal individual.

Once proper weight has been attained, the patient should follow the directions given below for the normal-weight diabetic.

IF THE PATIENT'S WEIGHT IS NORMAL

The diabetic's diet, like that of any individual, should be well balanced nutritionally and contain adequate amounts of protein, carbohydrates, fats, fruits, vegetables and minerals. Since, as explained earlier, the type of food has no bearing on diabetic control, no restrictions of this sort are necessary. But how many calories per day should the normal-weight diabetic consume?

Various formulas have been proposed for predicting the caloric requirements of individuals. Many physicians have been indoctrinated to speak of food prescribed to diabetics in terms of "grams per kilogram of body weight," but Dr. F. F. Davidoff points out the shortcomings of this method:

"It's so far removed that I've never learned the system myself. I've tried, but it just boggled my mind. And I don't think I should try to foist anything on patients that is so hard for me, particularly when cutting it that fine doesn't make much difference. It is my impression that only a minority of medical people still teach students to calculate food to the nearest few grams."[7]

The system of calculating calories strictly on weight has other fallacies as well: for one thing, a person requires progressively fewer calories with increasing age; for another, the patient's type of employment makes a difference. An athlete or manual laborer requires more food than a bookkeeper.

In the final analysis, the best guide to the proper caloric level of a diet is the indicator on the scale. From the very beginning, the patient should develop the habit of weekly or monthly weighings, and an increase or decrease in weight should dictate a like increase or decrease in calories.

The normal-weight patient, therefore, should simply make sure the diet he follows is well balanced nutritionally and keep a close eye on the scale. Anything more complicated than that is superfluous.

ADDITIONAL MEALS FOR THE DIABETIC
Food is also very important in counteracting the hypo-

glycemic effect of insulin and oral drugs. No matter which medication is used, a period of several hours without food may lower the blood sugar precariously, so it is strongly recommended that the patient eat something at regular intervals between meals.

Patients on regular insulin should snack two and one-half hours after the insulin injection, and those on intermediate insulins—NPH, Lente and Globin—should snack seven hours afterward. With oral drugs—Orinase, Diabinese, Dymelor, Tolinase, DBI—the patient should simply take something between meals and and at bedtime.

For prolonged effect, the mid-meal snack should consist primarily of protein and/or fat: carbohydrates simply do not last long enough.

DIABETIC FOODS

One of the ongoing dietary misconceptions is that of so-called "diabetic foods," caused by the assumption that carbohydrates are harmful, and resulting in many ingenious attempts to reduce the carbohydrate content of foods and sell them to the diabetic at excessive prices.

Aside from water-packed fruits which simply eliminate sugar solutions and syrup, these foods basically substitute a form of sugar that disintegrates more slowly for those foods which produce glucose—the so-called "harmful" sugar. These substitute sugars do *not* alter the caloric content of the diet—but obese diabetic patients draw the erroneous conclusion that as long as they use them, they are on the right track. Not so.

Also, many patients are convinced that because these ersatz foods cost more, they must be valuable. Again, not so. They are simply overpriced and, as far as the diabetic is concerned, useless.

The American Diabetes Association itself advises against the use of "diabetic foods" in its Exchange Diets, recommending instead that the diabetic select his food from the same sources used by other members of the family. I heartily concur.

ALCOHOL

In almost every diet prescribed for diabetic patients there appears the phrase "No alcoholic drinks," with no further explanation given. Patient and physician alike can only infer from this that alcohol somehow raises the blood sugar and affects diabetes adversely— but this is not true.

It *is* true that it wouldn't hurt the diabetic to stop drinking. One less imbiber of this deleterious drug would be beneficial all around. Unfortunately, most diabetics don't stop drinking and simply steal a drink here and there, feeling guilty all the time and convinced that they are doing themselves untold harm even while they are taking a quick one.

The fact is that the fate of alcohol in the human body is still a mystery. Its end products are carbon dioxide and water, and *not* sugar. It is true that some alcoholic beverages, such as beer and wine, contain sugar-producing substances, but even they have no greater ill-effects on diabetes than other carbohydrates which have been shown to be innocuous.

It is my custom to permit alcoholic beverages in moderation to all diabetics on a normal caloric diet. If the occasion calls for a little social drinking—then there's no reason not to enjoy yourself!

The Goodman "Meat Unlimited" Diet

BREAKFAST

Fruit, *See Fruit List below for portion and choice*
1 egg, hard-boiled, poached, scrambled, soft-boiled; prepare without butter
Toast, without crusts, 1 piece
Tea or coffee, without cream, sugar
Skim milk—8 ounces

LUNCH

Meat, poultry, or fish—large portion; *See Meat or Fish List.*
1 vegetable, *Vegetable List One*
1 salad, *Vegetable List One*

DINNER

Meat, poultry, or fish—large portion, *See Meat or Fish List.*
1 vegetable, *Vegetable List One or Two* (1 cup of fat-free vegetable soup or chicken soup may be substituted for 1 vegetable, *Vegetable List Two.*)
1 salad, *Vegetable List One*
Fruit—1 portion, *See Fruit List.*
Tea or coffee

EVENING

Skim milk or buttermilk—8 ounces.

Spices, vinegar, and low-calorie salad dressing may be used as desired. Vegetables are to be cooked in water or bouillon, no sauce or butter is to be added.

VEGETABLE LIST ONE
(1 measuring cup)

Artichoke, fresh	* Chicory or endive
Asparagus	Cucumbers
* Beet greens	* Dandelions
* Broccoli	Eggplant
Brussels Sprouts	* Escarole
Cabbage	Green Onions
* Carrot sticks, raw	* Kale
Cauliflower	* Leeks
Celery	Lettuce

* These vegetables contain large amounts of vitamin A. Use one each day.

Mushrooms
Okra
* Peppers
Radishes
Sauerkraut
* Spinach

Squash, Summer
String beans
* Swiss chard
* Tomatoes
* Water cress

VEGETABLE LIST TWO
(½ measuring cup)

Beets
* Carrots
Kohlrabi
Onions
Peas, small

* Pumpkin
Rutabaga
* Squash, winter
Turnips

FRESH FRUIT LIST
(Two portions daily)

Apple, small—1
Apricot, medium—2
Berries—1 cup
* Cantaloupe or watermelon—1 cup
Cherries—10–12
* Grapefruit, small—½
Grapes—15
* Lemon, lime, large—1
* Orange, small—1
Peach, medium—1
Pear, small—1
Pineapple—1 slice
Plum, medium—2
Prunes—3
* Tangerine, large—1

---

* These fruits contain large amounts of vitamin C. Use one each day.

MEAT LIST
(Any amount, boiled, broiled, or roasted)

Beef	Lamb
Brain	Liver
Chicken,	Turkey,
without skin	without skin
Kidney	Veal

FISH LIST
(Any amount, but no other kinds)

Carp	Perch
Cod, fresh or salt	Pike
Crabmeat	Scallops
Flounder	Shrimp
Haddock	Smelt
Halibut	Trout
Lobster	Whitefish
Oysters	

FREE
(The following foods may be eaten
any time, in any amount)

lean meat	coffee
fish	tea
poultry	clear bouillon
List One vegetables	low calorie soft
dill or sour pickles	drinks

5

MARRIAGE
AND CHILDREN

ONE NEED NOT HAVE a degree in psychiatry in order to be familiar with the painful emotional problems encountered by many young people as they mature, fall in love and begin to look ahead toward the possibility of marriage and their own families. The passions and confusions behind *Romeo and Juliet* are just as real today as they were when Shakespeare wrote about them.

Now add to this highly emotional period something such as diabetes. To someone in his late teens or early twenties, the announcement, almost always totally unexpected, that they are negatively different—that they must spend the rest of their lives dependent on injections and special regimentation—can be dangerously traumatic *unless* the announcement is accompanied by an honest picture of what diabetes is really like and the marvelous strides being taken.

All too often, however, the very opposite is true. The announcement of diabetes is accompanied by only a minimum of information or, worse, by distorted data and advice which, however well-intentioned, is totally out of date. Imagine what this means to those young adults:

"I was seventeen when they discovered I had diabetes," says Linda S., a very bright, attractive young woman. "I had already planned my life. I was going to attend a midwestern university, work as a reporter, travel a lot and then, hopefully, marry and have children." But the doctor's pronouncement, cold and impersonal, was like the voice of doom to Linda's plans. "I didn't think any man would want to marry someone with an incurable disease, and that's how I began to look at my illness—not as something that could be controlled, but as an incurable disease. I decided I would devote my life to a career only."

Another young woman, a secretary in an insurance office, found that the announcement of her condition made her feel like a criminal. "The way the whole thing was described, with needles and all that, made me picture myself like a drug addict. I felt guilty and dirty, and I didn't want anybody to find out about it. I knew I couldn't get married. I cried a lot, and I thought about suicide."

Even if the young diabetic is willing to keep an open mind about marriage, his or her parents may not be. Concerned not only for their child's physical well-being but also for the emotional damage they foresee as a result of diabetes, many parents become overprotective.

"My mom tried to turn me off of every girl I dated," says a young man whose diabetes was diagnosed only five days before his eighteenth birthday. "She was so afraid the girls would leave me flat when they found out about my being a diabetic that she tried to keep me from getting serious with anyone."

His mother admits that she interfered, but explains her feelings differently. "It wasn't just that the disease might be repugnant to the girls he liked, I worried that they wouldn't be willing to give my son the treatment he needed; to watch over him the way I was doing."

For most healthy-minded young people, the prospect of marriage is accompanied by the thought of raising one's own family. How does the advent of diabetes affect such considerations?

"I know my boyfriend would want children," said a young schoolteacher who, only recently diagnosed as a diabetic, was now reluctant to accept a marriage proposal. "I wouldn't want to fail him as a wife, and I've heard it's almost impossible for diabetic women to become pregnant. Would it be fair for me to marry him?"

And while this young teacher worried that she might not be able to become pregnant, her mother's fears were focused in precisely the opposite direction—on the complications which might ensue if her daughter *did* become pregnant. "A friend of mine had an aunt who was diabetic," the mother told me, "and she almost died during her pregnancy. There were all sorts of complications. And then the baby was oversized and they had to take it by caesarean."

Fears such as these do not stem solely from "old wives' tales." Many physicians themselves pass on similarly frightening information to their patients or even to other doctors. "Women with severe diabetes should be strongly advised to avoid pregnancy," Dr. Paul Beck told the Eighth Congress of the International Diabetes Federation meeting in Brussels.[1] Dr. Beck, an associate professor of medicine at the University of Colorado, stressed not only the possible complications of pregnancy but also warned against "adding to the genetic pool of diabetics" (passing diabetes on to one's offspring).

Of all the dogma surrounding marriage and childbearing for diabetics, there is probably none more well-entrenched than the "fact" that the disease is hereditary. "It's in our genes," a twenty-four-year-old bride told me tearfully. "My husband has it, and now we've found out my mother's sister had it too. We don't dare have children. And it's tearing our marriage apart."

In some cases, the marriage never takes place. A minister, finding out his daughter had diabetes, insisted she break off her engagement. "My wife and I feel guilty enough as it is," he explained. "We know diabetes is hereditary, so we are responsible for our daughter having it. That's terrible enough. We certainly don't want her doing the same thing to more kids. Marriage and children are out of the question."

One of the most depressing examples of misinformation is contained in the following statement made to a twenty-one-year-old college student. A gynecologist, upon discovering the student's diabetes in the course of a routine examination, immediately sat her down and volunteered this advice: "Since you have diabetes, you must carefully weigh the problems of marriage. You probably can't conceive. And if you do, there are all the dangers associated with pregnancy in diabetics —acidosis, hypertension, hydramnios and so on. If you should manage to overcome all these hazards, the baby probably will not live, or, if so, will be affected with congenital deformities."

Imagine that young lady's reaction to such an announcement. Before this, she had been psychologically well-adjusted to her diabetes, but now she was frightened. A friend suggested she seek another opinion, and so she came to me. I recall vividly how, on her first visit to my office, she sank into a chair, repeated what the gynecologist had told her and then looked me directly in the eye:

"Was he right, Dr. Goodman? Tell me the truth. I'm all worn out just thinking about it. I'm going with a young man and we're talking about marriage. What about having children?"

As is so often the case, my job with this young woman was not simply to "tell her the truth." In order to reopen the future she deserved, I had to spend many hours over many weeks and months undoing the psychic trauma inflicted on her by her gynecologist. To effect a "cure" of her diabetic neurosis, it was not enough to give her the true facts; I first had to explain the background which could have led her gynecologist to frighten her as he did.

The Background

All the authentic data show that diabetic females are normally fertile and can become pregnant as readily as nondiabetics. Why, then, would any doctor suggest the opposite? Was there a time when juvenile diabetics had difficulty conceiving?

The answer is, sadly, that there was a time when juvenile diabetic patients had difficulty doing anything at all. Before the availability of insulin (1921), pregnancy was almost unheard of in diabetic patients simply because they did not live long enough to conceive. The entire life span of the young adult with diabetes was usually limited to a few weeks or, at most, a few months. The question was not one of trying to help the young diabetic conceive, it was one of trying to help her live.

With the miraculous discovery of insulin by Banting and Best, the survival rates of young adults immediately began to increase. Long before physicians had achieved a full understanding of the best care for insulin-injecting patients, pregnancy became commonplace for young diabetics. But there were major problems.

It took time to gain an in-depth understanding of the best use of this new insulin, and even more time to farm out this information to the thousands of hospitals in the nation and the millions of doctors and diabetic patients. While this process of learning and dissemination took place, pregnant diabetics suffered frequently from episodes of ketoacidosis—an extreme type of excess acid condition which can lead to air-hunger and coma—and hypoglycemia. The mother's life was in constant jeopardy, to such a dramatic extent that her survival alone was hailed as a truly outstanding achievement.

It is this history, stemming from the immediate post-insulin period, that is the source of so many doctors' rusty stockpiles of misinformation. But times have changed. As diabetes research progressed, so too did the treatment of diabetic mothers. Each step forward in the understanding of diet and regimen was a step forward in the treatment of pregnant diabetics, and there was special research being done for them as well.

Pregnancy brings with it dramatic changes in many body functions, not the least of which is abnormal glucose readings even in many nondiabetic mothers. The regular injection of insulin amid such physical changes often produced unexpected results, but through trial and error and some exceptional clinical research, physicians rapidly improved their techniques. Soon, a relatively normal pregnancy for diabetics could be predicted with assurance.

Now, however, as the hazards to the diabetic mother moved off center stage, those of the offspring moved on. It quickly became apparent that many unfavorable events were taking place in the fetuses of diabetic mothers. Most striking was the inordinately high mortality rate. Then the records began to show fetuses of excessively large size and weight, and organs—heart, kidneys and so on—that were oversized and congenital deformities. The offspring were generally described as "big, fat and full-faced." Full term, they often weighed more than ten pounds, and even premature they weighed seven to nine pounds, due not to excessive accumulation of fluid (edema) but to actual fleshiness and increased length.

Babies of diabetic mothers were, without question, sick babies. There was great danger of prematurity, early respiratory distress, hypoglycemia (usually developing within six hours after birth), congenital malformations, birth trauma and infection.[2]

This situation held extraordinarily depressing prospects for potential parents. Physicians valiantly sought answers to alleviate their anguish, but in the meantime obstetricians reached agreement that the large babies were poor candidates for normal delivery. It seemed wise, they reasoned, to remove the oversized babies after thirty-six to thirty-eight weeks, thus obviating difficult labor and taking the infant while life was still strong.

This became a generally accepted routine everywhere, even after the exchange of data clearly showed the offspring were still dying postpartum, usually as a result of hyaline membrane disease (respiratory failure). Eventually, it was discovered that the prematurity associated with early delivery was, in itself, the greatest hazard for all of these children.

Meanwhile, research continued. The first major breakthrough occurred at the Joslin Clinic when Dr. Priscilla White reported a hormone imbalance in pregnant diabetic women. Dr. White organized a special clinic where she could study this condition, and where, under her personal supervision, diabetic mothers were separated from others and given special care and treatment, including the administration of estrogen and progesterone.

The result was a surprisingly improved survival rate, but the greatest surprise of all proved to be the true reason for Dr. White's success. Thanks to a subsequent study of pregnant diabetics by Drs. Black and Miller, it became apparent that the survival rate was due not to the administration of hormones, but rather to the all-around improvement in diabetic treatment the mothers received: greater consistency in technique, more concern with special diet, careful scheduling of insulin injections, proper courses of exercise, etc. The secret of normal pregnancy and childbirth for the diabetic mother had proven to be unexpectedly simple: the careful control of the mother's diabetes.

Additional documentation was provided by the Hopkins Group headed by Dr. John E. Tyson. Based on the excellent results they obtained, Dr. Tyson and his colleagues could report: "In patients with *well-controlled* diabetes, perinatal mortality is negligible. This prospective study documents that preterm delivery is unnecessary. . . . Vaginal delivery at term is not only possible but preferable *when gestational diabetes is well-controlled*."[8]

In Dr. Tyson's group, this control was such that glucose values were consistently kept below 100 mg./ 100 ml., and this was accomplished entirely by restricting caloric intake, thereby confining weight gain to less than eight ounces per week. Using this regimen, there were no intrauterine or neonatal deaths, no increase in perinatal mortality or morbidity as the fetus grew, and only minimal complications during delivery.

Dr. Tyson and his associates proved that it was not diabetes itself that was the culprit but, rather, extreme, prolonged fluctuations in glucose readings—in order words, *badly controlled* diabetes. Freed from the burden of these conditions, none of the babies developed significant complications, congenital malformations or respiratory distress syndromes.

I heartily agree that the fate of the fetus is tied directly to the degree of diabetes control achieved during pregnancy. In my office, I have a photograph album filled with snapshots of the children of numerous diabetic patients. These pictures have been collected over the past twenty-five years, and thanks to the careful control of the mothers' diabetes during pregnancy, all of these snapshots show normal, healthy, vigorous children.

Today, because of constantly improving techniques, we can look forward confidently to a normal baby, delivered in normal fashion at full term by a healthy, well-regulated diabetic mother.

Heredity

In 1973, Dr. D. L. Rimoin, distinguished professor of
pediatrics and medicine at the University of California
at Los Angeles, stated in no uncertain terms that the
World Health Organization had been wrong in 1965
when, in order to avoid "adding to the genetic pool of
diabetics," it counseled against diabetics marrying and
having children.[4]

I concur wholeheartedly with Dr. Rimoin. My personal clinical experience over many years has convinced me there is no proven hereditary basis for diabetes. Of the diabetic parents I have known who have
one or more offspring, not a single child—not one—
has developed diabetes. Conversely, a review of the
diabetic children I have treated over more than twenty-
five years fails to uncover even one parent with diabetes!

Still, as shown earlier, far too many doctors continue to voice the out-of-date theory that diabetes is
hereditary. Only infrequently are diabetic patients
encouraged to proceed normally in raising a family. Far
more often, they are warned that they will very likely
be passing on their handicap to their children. How
did such a misconception arise?

The cornerstone of this theory is the frequent occurrence of diabetes in similar twins when one of them
has the disease. Elliott Joslin analyzed this incidence in
thirty-three sets of similar twins and sixty-three pairs
of dissimilar twins, Hildegard Berg studied forty-six
similar twins and Friedrich Umber worked with nineteen pairs. Although these samples were far too small
to provide statistically meaningful data, dangerously
broad inferences were drawn from the studies. The
medical profession decided—and so advised the public—that diabetes was a hereditary disease and that

children inherited diabetes according to the Mendelian Law as a recessive characteristic.

This offered frightening prospects for diabetic parents. If diabetes were, as these physicians suggested, an autosomal recessive disease, the risk of diabetes in the offspring of diabetic parents would be considerable. Where only one of the parents was diabetic, one out of four children would be expected to have diabetes, and where both parents were diabetic, *three* out of four children would be likely to inherit the disease.

Today, as Dr. Rimoin rightly points out, the concept of recessive inheritance can be overturned very easily: by simply noting the studies that have proven diabetes in the children of two diabetic parents to be too infrequent to support such a theory. The statistically meaningful studies Dr. Rimoin cites for support are far from isolated examples. D. A. Pyke's investigation also revealed that the incidence of diabetes in the children of two diabetics is far lower than would be predicted if the disease were inherited as a single recessive gene.[5] The same is true for Joslin's 1959 data and a 1966 English study. Mendelian Law simply does not apply to diabetes.

But if the disease is not hereditary, how are we to explain the frequent occurrence in similar twins when one of them has the disease? And what about the recent data indicating diabetes occurring more frequently in some families than one would expect from chance alone? A 1968 Canadian study indicates a two- to fourfold increase in diabetes among the brothers and sisters of diabetics above forty years of age. The study also shows a four- to fivefold increase when onset for the diabetic occurred between the ages of twenty and thirty-nine, and a ten- to fourteenfold increase when onset occurred before the age of twenty. From studies such as these, it appears that brothers and sisters in any family are more likely to have diabetes if any one member has the disease, and that this possibility increases the younger the member is at the onset.

Without questioning the accuracy of this data, I must point out that it offers no evidence whatsoever about the likelihood of diabetic parents passing on the disease to their offspring. What it does show is that a husband and wife, *regardless of whether or not they have diabetes,* may have in their gene package some unique combination which tends to produce diabetic children.

What is this unique gene combination? We do not know, and finding out may very well be a long, drawn-out process. Dr. James V. Neel, professor of human genetics at the University of Michigan, has called diabetes "a geneticist's nightmare."[6] There are three basic reasons why.

First, due to the great variability in clinical manifestations, there is substantial disagreement as to what actually constitutes a diabetic, as to where the dividing line should be drawn between the disease and "normality." Dr. Neel, for example, would restrict the interpretation to those cases where there are, or are expected to be, pathological consequences. Other physicians disagree. It is because of such differences that figures showing the incidence of diabetes differ so widely from study to study. Consider this data:

A diabetic survey in England (1962) reported the frequency of known diabetics as two percent in those over seventy years of age, but the U.S. National Health Survey (1960) reported an incidence of double that (four percent) for persons in the same age group. Meanwhile, a large-scale survey in Georgia found abnormal glucose tolerance (one "definition" of diabetes) in 7.4 percent of persons over seventy, while another study of a thousand largely ambulatory patients over sixty not known to have diabetes found 8.8 percent with diabetes or "potential diabetes." And in a study conducted by the University of Michigan in Tecumseh, a Michigan community of over seven thousand population, it was found that at least twenty percent of the people over forty fulfilled one definition for "potential diabetes," the attainment of hyperglycemic levels one hour after a standard glucose load.

The second problem which makes diabetes a "geneticist's nightmare," is the fact that the disease becomes more frequent with age, thus making cross-sectional studies in time totally unrepresentative of the true picture. Add to this the tremendous variability in the age of onset within the two major categories—juvenile and adult—and the fact that juvenile diabetes is entirely different from the adult form, and you have considerable confusion.

The third problem is that of rapidly changing environment. We have good reason to suspect that a modern industrial society offers living conditions, such as overnutrition and underactivity, which are very important to the onset of diabetes—but which change so rapidly that statistics based on one generation may not be applicable to the next.

It is these kinds of very practical problems which will make a full understanding of diabetic genetics extremely difficult to achieve. Meanwhile, the abnormally low incidence of the disease in the children of diabetic parents, and in the parents of diabetic children, is sufficient to enable us to stop torturing young diabetics with the fear of passing on the disease to their unborn children.

Which returns us finally to where we began this chapter—with the story of Linda S., the bright, attractive young lady who, having been coldly advised of her diabetes at age seventeen, determined to give up all thoughts of marriage and family.

"I decided to follow the advice of my school counselor; I sought psychiatric help. After two years of therapy, I finally believed that diabetes need not be fatal . . . Then I met Steven. I knew after several months of dating him that I cared about him very much. I felt he cared about me, too. He knew about my diabetes, but it didn't seem to matter to him. Soon, Steven proposed . . .

"Steven confided in me that he had his doubts about having children, but after reading about diabetes, these doubts cleared up. I also spoke to my doctor about having children, and he assured me there should be no difficulty in conceiving or keeping my diabetes under control during pregnancy or delivery.

"After a year of marriage, we decided to have a child. In my own mind, and Steven's too, I was prepared to have a healthy baby.

"Arlen Mark was four years old in April, and I still can't believe how lucky I was. Yes, it is possible for a diabetic to marry, to have children, and most of all, to lead a normal, healthy life."

6

COMPLICATIONS

No one expects the patient or his family to react happily to the news that he has diabetes. It is a very serious business and must be treated accordingly. However, odd as it may sound, there *are* positive aspects to the disease, and it is important for the patient and his family to know about them. It is not only unnecessary, but dangerous—physically, emotionally and psychologically—to focus constantly only on the hazards of diabetes, and nowhere is this truer than with the question of medical complications. Here, the shouts from some doctors and diabetic journals are much like the cry of "Fire!" in a crowded theater: the warning can be far more dangerous than the condition it concerns.

A positive, healthy attitude is vital to the best control of diabetes, as it is with almost any serious disease. Yet how is the diabetic to attain such an outlook when he is bombarded by fearful warnings about almost certain gangrene, amputation, blindness, heart attacks and other dreadful afflictions?

"I didn't know too much about diabetes," says L.N., an automotive engineer, "but after it showed up in my examination, I read a couple of books about it. I wish I hadn't! Diabetes is bad enough, but all that stuff it can lead to is terrifying. The business about infection nearly wrecked me. I was afraid to leave the house because I might pick up germs or cut myself or something."

Unfortunately, such alarming books are the rule rather than the exception, even those which, from their titles, one would expect to help the diabetic adjust to his disease. For example, when the recent book, *Counseling and Rehabilitating the Diabetic,* by John Cull and Richard Hardy, was reviewed by the American Diabetes Association, the article called the chapter on psychological adjustment to functional loss a "negative approach" which, because it equated *all* diabetes with the crippling aspects of the disease, would "merely create or provoke anxiety."[1]

With nothing to offset a frighteningly negative picture of the future, the diabetic and his family often react with enormous alarm to the first sign of some new "symptom" —a pain, for instance. When a diabetic develops neuropathy (nerve damage), entire families, all well-versed in horror stories, accompany the patient en masse to the doctor's office to find out what dire complication this pain is leading to. In actual fact, diabetic neuropathy indicates no permanent complication at all. Rather, it is connected in some still unexplained manner with the deranged metabolism of unregulated diabetes and heals soon after good diabetic control has been achieved and maintained. This fact notwithstanding, patients and their families are so inculcated with fear of complications that to them the pain means the onset of some horrible new complication for sure—so much so that whenever a patient with diabetic neuropathy comes into my office, I alert my staff and household to be prepared for a galaxy of phone calls, local and long distance, from members of the patient's family.

Other types of pain produce similar results. I recall a very frightened twenty-six-year-old girl who consulted me in despair about her leg pains. Her mother had heard that diabetics "always lose their legs," so she was certain the pains represented the first stage of the process.

In reality, they were caused by diabetic neuritis which, although painful, disappears completely after the diabetes is brought under control. The emotional pain this young woman and her family suffered before the true situation was explained to them was needless.

No pain was needed to frighten nineteen-year-old Ted L. His fear arose from an episode in a television series titled *Medical Center*. "The show was about a diabetic going blind," Ted told me. "And the doctor was using a laser to try and preserve vision a little longer."

That program reminded Ted that he had heard a great deal about diabetics going blind. "People are always telling me about diabetic friends who've lost their eyesight. It's starting to get me uptight. And now it's on TV. I don't think I can handle it." Typically, the television show failed to point out that the great majority of diabetics who have carefully controlled their disease suffer no visual impairment whatsoever—and that there are many medical advances available to those who do.

Television doctors, however, are not the only ones who cause unnecessary alarm. One of my patients consulted an ear, nose and throat specialist for paralysis of a vocal cord. Unable to think of any other reason for the paralysis, the doctor blamed the patient's diabetes! The real cause proved to be quite different. A well-regulated diabetic, such as this patient was, rarely if ever develops a neurologic complication . . . but the doctor found diabetes a short road to a simple answer.

Another patient of mine, visiting a dermatologist, asked him to inspect a lesion on her leg. The doctor asked, "Do you have diabetes?" When she acknowledged she did, he stated unequivocally, "This is a diabetic lesion." Immediately, the woman was petrified. Would she lose her leg?

The truth was the lesion in question was *not* caused

by diabetes and, even if it had been, there would have been no need for concern over it. Diabetic skin lesions do not produce serious complications and usually heal completely in due time.

Dentists, too, are often guilty of frightening patients by implying that normal dental procedures may have abnormal results in the case of the diabetic. One of my patients, for example, was told, following extensive peridontal surgery, that the deterioration of his gums had been due to diabetes in the first place and, therefore, the dentist "couldn't guarantee that the procedure would be successful." Neither statement was correct.

The tendency to overemphasize the importance of diabetes is commonplace among hospital personnel, a factor which adds to the distress of the diabetic patient already overwrought by the illness that prompted his admission. A young man I know was admitted to a hospital for the diagnosis and eventual removal of a lung due to a probable lung tumor. His life was in jeopardy, but after several days of harassment by the house staff and other attendants about his diabetes control, he asked me:

"Dr. Goodman, I thought I was sent to the hospital for my lung condition. It seems like everybody here is concerned only about my diabetes which I know is well-controlled and causing me no difficulty. Why all the excitement about this? Have they forgotten why I entered the hospital?"

Why the great concern? Because all of them had been taught that no medical or surgical condition will progress satisfactorily unless the diabetic patient has a normal blood sugar and negative urine tests—a goal calling for constant checks of blood and urine sugar. When, as is often the case, this ideal state cannot be achieved, even when their diabetes is well-controlled (see Chapter Three), it becomes a source of great frustration to all concerned—a frustration which cannot be hidden from an already overanxious patient.

Such fears are not limited to patients in the hospital environment. "They say I could lose control of my diabetes even if I get just a virus of some sort," a young housewife told me. "I'm not a worrywart, but that really shook me up. I know that if I lose control it could mean diabetic coma. All just because I caught a virus from somebody. How do I live a normal life with that on my mind?"

The family of this young woman had been seriously affected by this concern. "Our house has become as sterile as a hospital," her husband told me. "The kids and I worry about where we go and who we see. All of us are becoming hypochondriacs. And if, God forbid, we do catch something—a sore throat maybe—we not only worry, we feel guilty as the devil. It's hurting all of us."

Such an atmosphere can be a traumatic experience for children with a parent or brother or sister who is diabetic. They are not only deprived of a home-like environment but denied sympathy when they themselves become sick.

Even a constant focus on a germ-free environment is not enough to satisfy the fears of many unreasonably alarmed diabetics. "My concern is I haven't been able to discover any concrete steps to prevent those complications I read about," one patient told me. "I've asked my doctor about this, and he says the important thing is to keep my blood sugar at the proper levels on a day-to-day basis. As long as I do this, I'm told, the complications probably won't develop. But that isn't enough. I feel I ought to be doing something specific to avoid complications. And, also, I've heard that some diabetics have complications even though they do everything they're supposed to."

Such continuing frustration sometimes causes the diabetic to make a complete about-face. Deciding that there is really nothing he can do, that the onslaught of crippling complications is inevitable, he gives up, throws caution to the wind and fails to heed even the most elementary rules of prevention. The result is a foregone conclusion.

The most tragic thing about all this is the total lack of necessity. A physician's duty is to provide patients with enough information to cope with their future, but he is certainly under no obligation to frighten them with lurid speculative descriptions. Such dire warnings serve only to make the patients vulnerable to a host of imaginary ailments, while blinding them and their families to the positive aspects of their situation. What are these aspects?

In simplest terms, a diabetic may be compared to a man who has been in a serious car accident and survives. The brush with death may cause him to begin developing good safety habits toward the prevention of another accident: good auto maintenance, fastening his seat belt, staying within the speed limit, obeying other laws of the road.

In the same way, the diabetic can benefit from his disorder by developing good health habits, not only for his diabetes control, but for his general health as well: sufficient rest, no smoking, exercise, good foot care, balanced diet, moderate drinking, and, perhaps most important of all, a thorough medical examination at regular intervals. Such a regimen gives the diabetic a significant health *advantage* over most other people.

Another positive aspect is that the patient and his family establish a system of twenty-four-hours-a-day, seven-days-a-week contact with his doctor. I instruct my patients to phone me at the first sign of any possible symptom, regardless of the hour, for I much prefer to get a telephone call at three in the morning when a problem can be treated at home than to get one at nine in the morning from the hospital emergency room. The value of such a "hot-line" system cannot be overestimated, and it gives the diabetic another significant advantage over most nondiabetics.

A final advantage is knowledge. All human beings ought to understand their bodies better, to know their strengths and limitations, to understand what poses a real danger and what does not, but few people do. They lack the incentive to undertake such a study. The diabetic (and his family) have that incentive.

In supplying such knowledge to my patients, I have found that it is important not only to tell them the facts about each possible area of medical complication, but also, wherever possible, to explain the background which may have led to any distorted information they received.

That is what I will do in the remainder of this chapter.

Infection

No area of possible complication is more destructive to the family life of the diabetic than fear of infection. The unnatural strain such a concern places upon the nondiabetic members of the family can result in a wide variety of psychological problems—guilt, frustration, a feeling of being unloved, anger toward the diabetic—yet no other area of possible complication is more firmly entrenched than the belief that diabetics have a predilection to infection. The diabetic learns this early, from other patients, from books and articles, even from many doctors and nurses—yet such is *not* the case.

Authorities with the stature of Dr. M. D. Siperstein of the University of California are not only impressed with the resistance of diabetics to infection, they state categorically that diabetics are no more susceptible to infection than other individuals.[2] Dr. Siperstein has seen diabetics with severe ulcers of the skin come to his clinic for years without developing infection, and he is convinced that much of the problem lies not with any abnormal predilection to infection but rather with something as relatively (and unfortunately) common as too-frequent catheterization of the urinary bladder.

Despite such authoritative testimony, the erroneous belief still prevails—and again the basis lies in history. Prior to the discovery of insulin, diabetics had good reason to fear infections: tuberculosis, for instance, was the rampant "great killer" at the turn of the century, and diabetics were particularly susceptible; carbuncles and related inflammations called furuncles (boils) were commonplace; many other such afflictions besieged the diabetic.

Today these infections are rare and diabetics suffer from them no more than nondiabetics. This is certainly due in part to the effective results of modern drug therapy, but there is another reason as well—the improved physical status of the diabetic himself, as a result of insulin and other measures, has made the patients more resistant to these as well as to all other infections, with very rare exceptions.

There is a secondary basis for the diabetic's fear of infection. It is commonly thought that infection destroys the control of diabetes, thus predisposing the patient to ketoacidosis and diabetic coma, and endangering his very life. He is taught that infection, trauma, stress or drugs will cause peripheral insulin resistance which requires more insulin, that his blood sugar and insulin requirement will increase during illness, that if he doesn't meet the increased demand for insulin, he will very possibly get hyperglycemia.[8]

To complete this terrifying picture, he is often taught that the deterioration of his diabetic control may show up initially as an elevation of the blood sugar, so the moment he feels the slightest bit ill, the diabetic performs the urine tests and, sure enough, there are the glucose and acetone! Immediately, he is certain he will soon wind up in the hospital.

All this is *unnecessary*. The properly informed diabetic need not be concerned about his ability to ward off loss of control and ketoacidosis in the face of illness. He need only continue taking his full insulin dose while making certain he consumes and retains an adequate amount of carbohydrate.

If the illness produces loss of appetite or nausea, the diabetic can usually maintain his carbohydrate intake by consuming sweetened fruit juices, cold soft drinks, soup and crackers, gelatin desserts and other carbohydrates on a frequent basis. This procedure will also prevent hypoglycemic reactions.

If there is vomiting, the frequent consumption (every one or two hours) of high carbohydrate drinks—orange juice, tea with sugar, etc.—will usually handle the matter, but if vomiting persists to the point where the patient is unable to retain even these liquids, then it is essential that he contact his doctor who can see to it that the patient is administered glucose intravenously, preferably in the hospital. This points up the importance of the "hot line" mentioned earlier. It is vital that the diabetic always be able to contact his physician.

My rules for diabetics who become ill can be summarized as follows:

1. Be sure to take the usual insulin dose.
2. Eat regular meals as much as possible.
3. If unable to eat solid food, or after vomiting, take orange juice, ginger ale or other carbohydrate liquids hourly.
4. If vomiting persists, keep in constant touch with your physician.

Wound healing

Wound healing is a related area, and, again, many physicians are convinced that the diabetic heals poorly and the uncontrolled diabetic even more so. Yet I have not encountered any scientific studies to substantiate this concept.

On the other hand, I *can* recall an important study reported in 1942 by Dr. Greene of Iowa City, who compared the healing rate of surgical wounds of diabetics and nondiabetics. His study clearly showed that wounds healed as well in the diabetic as in the normal individual. Most impressive was the finding that those diabetics with the highest blood sugars healed most rapidly of all!

Dr. Greene, recognizing that the lower extremities of the human body present a special situation which predisposes to slow healing irrespective of diabetic control, excluded these areas from his study. He was absolutely correct. There are certain factors, still unexplained, which delay healing in the lower third of the legs and in the feet of normal persons—and this is *equally* true of the diabetic and the nondiabetic.

It is fair to state that under equivalent conditions, the diabetic can and does heal as rapidly as the normal individual.

Atherosclerosis

To the layman, many popularized articles appear to offer "proof" that diabetes is the cause of atherosclerosis, the underlying lesion of heart disease and stroke. The truth is, however, that atherosclerosis is the leading cause of death in the United States in *nondiabetics* as well as diabetics. Heart disease can strike anyone. To take just one example, numerous fatal heart attacks were reported from Vietnam in soldiers in their twenties, none of whom had diabetes.

The actual cause of atherosclerosis and its resultant heart disease is not yet known. Why, then, burden the diabetic and his family with the fear that his disorder will lead inevitably to a heart attack? For other scare stories, see also the notes for this chapter regarding the recent controversy on the drug tolbutamide.[4]

Without question, it is important to know that there is a statistical association between atherosclerosis and diabetes. Heart disease accounts for over half of the deaths among diabetics, and in a study of fifty thousand fatalities, coronary heart disease was reported in about twice as many diabetic as nondiabetic men and in three times as many diabetic women. It is a serious business and must be considered seriously. Armed with this information, however, the diabetic can take those measures that can help preserve his life.

First, he must maintain proper control of his diabetes. Many diabetic specialists, including myself, are firmly convinced that precise diabetic control can forestall the development of vascular lesions, and everyone agrees that *poor* control is bad. J. M. Moss found, for example, that patients in poor diabetic control showed a ten percent decrease in longevity.[5,6]

Second, the diabetic should present himself for thorough examination at least once a year. In this way, should any complication develop it would be detected immediately, and properly treated.

In sum, atherosclerosis is certainly a complication the diabetic should be careful of, but in *no* way does having diabetes mean that heart disease is inevitable, and it must be remembered that atherosclerosis is the leading cause of deaths in the United States among diabetics and nondiabetics alike. It picks no favorites. The diabetic who maintains excellent control of his diabetes through total adherence to his prescribed regimen of diet, exercise and good habits, and through thorough periodical examinations by his physician, will help himself immeasurably.

Diabetic neuropathy

A complication already mentioned is neuropathy (nerve damage). This is one of the most frequent and distressing ailments associated with diabetes, but it can be treated effectively simply my maintaining good diabetic control, and, here again, the greatest danger is from the patient's fears running rampant. It usually attacks the lower extremities, though all the peripheral and autonomic nerves of the body are susceptible, and is characterized by destruction of the protective (myelin) sheath, much like the damaged insulation of an electric light cord, leaving the nerve exposed.

The symptom which brings the patient to the physician is pain—pain and paresthesias (tingling sensations) of all gradations of discomfort, from feelings of numbness, crawling and tingling, to extreme sensitivity even to the bed sheets, to steady or darting pains. All of these symptoms are worse at night and lead the patient to envision a multitude of serious illnesses such as stroke or cancer. By the time the doctor is consulted, not only is the patient terribly agitated, but his entire family as well.

The most important thing a doctor can do at this time is to explain over and over again to the patient and his family the nature and progress of this painful condition; to make the point that the marked discomfort is *not* caused by a fatal, serious disease but is brought on by uncontrolled diabetes; and to assure them that the nerve damage will begin to heal once good control of the diabetes has been achieved and maintained for a reasonable period.

Although the pain may extend for a period of weeks or even months, it will be handled much more easily when all concerned understand that it emanates from a

benign condition—and is unlikely to bother the diabetic
again.

Eyesight

Many press releases and news articles emphasize the
blinding aspects of diabetes, often implying that a condition called retinopathy is inevitable if the patient has
diabetes long enough. Ophthalmologists who support
the view that diabetic patients are predestined to lose
their eyesight also maintain that good or poor control
of diabetes makes no difference.

*Such opinions are dangerous and based on limited
or out-of-date experience.* Retinopathy is by no means
"predestined." The firmly held viewpoint of diabetic
specialists with large clinical experience is that such
damage is dependent on the course of the diabetes—
the better the diabetic control, the less the incidence
and possibility of retinal lesions.

The concept that blindness was inevitable for the
diabetic arose during those years before good overall
control of diabetes (diet, exercise, oral medication, insulin, etc.) was properly understood. During this time,
it became evident to the medical profession that an-
atomic abnormalities were occurring in the small blood
vessels of diabetics.

Put simply, diabetes is capable of damaging the
capillaries in the retina, causing them to weaken and
bleed. If the condition progresses, new blood vessels
may form on the surface of the retina and in the
vitreous humor in the center of the eye, causing further
hemorrhages and blurred vision. In some cases, the
blood is reabsorbed and the vision clears. In other
cases, the hemorrhage causes scar tissue which may
then contract, pulling the retina, detaching or tearing
it, and thereby resulting in permanent blindness.

This is a hazard which the knowledgeable diabetic

should very clearly understand, but he should also understand what the latest developments in proper diabetic care can do to prevent or delay such occurrences. Many current studies strongly emphasize the importance of good diabetic control, as we have discussed throughout the book, on problems regarding eyesight. For instance, a twenty-five-year study reported in *The Sight-Saving Review,* involving four thousand patients and a computer analysis of over one million pieces of information, clearly showed that retinopathy appeared to be significantly influenced by both the duration and degree of diabetic control.[7]

My personal experience supports this view. Continuous, excellent control of diabetes tends to prevent damage to retinal capillaries. I have actually seen cases of advanced retinopathy disappear when a patient converted from poor to good diabetic control.

Even with retinopathy, however, there are many other weapons—an amazingly wide variety of procedures, many newly available—for the preservation of vision. The laser, for example.

An intense beam of light is directed into the retina and focused on a tiny spot, in a process that may be compared with focusing the sun's rays through a magnifying glass to burn a hole in a leaf. Heat energy generated by the light produces a small burn which destroys the retinopathy by coagulating weakened blood vessels or destroying the proliferating vessels. If there are fragile new vessels in the treated area, they can also be destroyed, thereby preventing serious bleeding. The burn heals as a scar.

This process, called photocoagulation, was first used in 1955, and can be done with a xenon arc photocoagulator, an argon laser, a ruby laser or any combination of these instruments. The xenon arc lamp generates an intense beam of white light and was the first device used in this treatment, but the most recent development has been the argon laser which has a fine green beam and can be very accurately focused and controlled.

While vision is occasionally improved, this procedure is actually designed to prevent the more serious consequences of diabetic retinopathy and to maintain the vision at its pretreatment level. The aim is to protect the patient's most important central vision while sacrificing, if necessary, some of his less important side vision. Fortunately, the abnormal new vessels rarely grow over the essential part of the retina, called the macula, necessary for central and reading vision.

There can be no doubt that the results achieved so far with photocoagulation have been most rewarding, and it is already in use in clinics and doctors' offices across the nation. In addition, the National Eye Institute, part of HEW's National Institutes of Health, is supporting a nationwide study involving sixteen cooperating medical centers to further evaluate the process. The sponsors are optimistic that the study will furnish even more valuable information.

There is even new hope for those who are actually blind from massive vitreous hemorrhage or retinal detachment. Vitrectomy, a new type of operation performed under the microscope, is saving the sight of some patients. Dr. Guy O'Grady reported at the annual South Western Diabetes Symposium, sponsored by the Diabetes Association of Southern California, that he was able to produce a significant benefit in patients with a new surgical device called a vitreous infusion suction cutter, developed at the Bascom Palmer Eye Institute.[8] Looking like a large metal syringe, the extractor is powered by a small electric motor and contains three concentric tubes in its head, enabling the surgeon to incise, remove the vitreous material by suction, release bands causing retinal detachment and infuse saline solution.

Dr. O'Grady estimates that about fifty percent of the patients currently blind from diabetic retinopathy are candidates for this operation, and of the group already operated on, about half have been helped significantly. Dr. Robert D. Reinecke, ophthalmology chairman at Albany Medical College, says that there may be twenty-five thousand candidates for vitrectomy in the U.S., including patients with end-stage diabetic retinopathy who cannot be treated with laser therapy.[9] The results which may be achieved with this procedure are strikingly depicted in an article in the *Cleveland Plain Dealer*:

> Henry A. Gearing, 52, of Parma, is coming home tomorrow from California with newly restored vision in his left eye. Gearing has been blind for six months from blood clots in his eyes caused by diabetes. He was operated on September 30 at the Stanford University Medical Center with a new technique to remove such clots. . . . His bandages were removed in 24 hours, and it was very dramatic for him and his family. He could see. . . . He walked into the hospital with a cane and walked out last Friday with no assistance.[10]

As dramatically impressive as these results are, I still wish to make it clear that, first, being a diabetic does *not* mean you have to go through any of this, and, second, that even every diabetic with retinopathy need not suffer visual impairment. All opthalmologists have had the happy experience of discovering diabetic retinopathy only to have the patient's eyesight remain good. Blind persons constitute a very small proportion indeed of the total diabetic population—and that is the experience of all diabetic specialists.

Dental complications

There is a widespread belief among dentists, a concept unfortunately supported by many physicians, that the diabetic has an increased predilection to various dental hazards—caries, peridontal involvement, etc.—which result in the loss of teeth. Even when performing essential procedures for a diabetic, procedures unhesitatingly undertaken for nondiabetic persons, fear lurks in the dentist's mind that somehow the outcome won't turn out normally, and he conveys this fear to the patient.

The belief has *no* modern basis in fact and could be injurious to the patient's general good health. Some years ago, Dr. Jack Samuels and his associates undertook an impartial study in the Mt. Sinai Hospital Diabetes Clinic in Cleveland, Ohio, and found that the diabetic was in no way more susceptible to dental ills than anyone else, given adequate dental attention. The dentist—and his patient—need have no fear.

Kidney damage

Kidney damage ("nephropathy") is a very serious condition for diabetics and nondiabetics alike. It occurs in only a small percentage of diabetics, and in a still smaller percentage of those who consistently practice good diabetic control. When the disease does occur, it presents extremely serious complications, whether the patient is diabetic or not, in its most advanced stage even resulting in death. Short of that drastic result, however, there is still considerable room for optimism.

There is, first of all, the opportunity for transplants. Dr. Michall J. Kussman of the Joslin Clinic points out that diabetics with renal transplants have a two-and-a-half times better survival rate than do others who have suffered kidney damage.[11]

There is also dialysis. At a symposium on end-stage diabetic nephropathy sponsored by the National Institute of Arthritis, Metabolism and Digestive Disease, Dr. Constantine Hampers stated that the results of dialysis on diabetic patients were immensely better than any previously reported. At the end of the first years of dialysis, over three-quarters of the juvenile-type diabetics and almost two-thirds of the adult-type diabetics had survived the procedure[12]—compare this with the fact that a few years before, diabetic kidney patients were considered too hopeless even to put on dialysis! In addition, almost half of the juvenile-type patients and over half of the adult-type patients were able to return to their jobs, a basis for rehabilitation considered very good in kidney patients. And this was in 1974—medicine has advanced even more since then.

Once again, with nephropathy as with other aspects of health, good diabetic control is a key to good health —but even with the small percentage of diabetics who do develop kidney damage, the continued advances in medical technology offer a good deal of hope.

Foot lesions

One of the pervading fears of the diabetic and his family is the firm conviction that he is destined to lose one or both legs. From news articles, television programs, other patients he meets in waiting rooms, "helpful" friends and relatives, even some doctors and nurses, the diabetic is made to feel that the feet and legs are areas of great potential trouble. All too quickly he begins to envision prolonged hospitalization, loss of limb and even premature death. From this point, it is only a short step to an hysterical fear of leaving his bed or his chair.

Such psychological pain is totally unnecessary, for three very good reasons. First, loss of limb is not some overnight process. (Except in the case of a sudden thrombosis, which diabetics are no more prone to than nondiabetics.) It takes place in many stages, the first being the development of a diabetic foot lesion as the result of nerve damage. As we have seen, such neuropathy arises from poor diabetes control, and so the *properly* controlled diabetic should have no fear of nerve damage or foot lesions.

When nerve damage, from poor control, does occur, it may result in muscle imbalance that produces deformities of the toes and feet. This condition, in turn, leads to abnormal pressure in certain areas of the feet such as the metatarsal arch, and excessive callus formation which impinges upon the underlying skin. When these factors combine with the extreme fragility of the tissue, the groundwork is present for skin damage and ulcer formation.

Many authorities (and much of the general public) believe that foot lesions in diabetics are the result of poor arterial circulation. This is not true. While it is a fact that many older diabetics have an inadequate blood flow in their feet as a result of atherosclerosis, this has nothing to do with lesions, and, in fact, there is usually quite enough flow to promote healing, provided the patient remains off his feet continuously.

The second principal reason for not worrying about foot lesions is that even for the susceptible diabetic—one who has peripheral nerve damage—such foot lesions are entirely preventable by employing proper foot hygiene and the services of a podiatrist well-versed in diabetic foot care.

The podiatrist, by training, skillful technique and experience, has the necessary expertise to prevent injury to the skin. The podiatrist who knows about the foot problems of the diabetic trims calluses and nails—the elderly nerve-damaged diabetic should *not* trim his own toenails, corns and calluses—instructs the patient in proper foot hygiene and, when necessary, fits prostheses and special shoes to alleviate pressure in crucial areas of the feet.

Third, even if a lesion *should* develop on the foot of a diabetic, prompt treatment brings about rapid and complete healing. In order to accomplish this, the patient must keep off his feet entirely for twenty-four hours each day with the lesion exposed to the air. Better yet, the lesion dries up and heals more rapidly under a cradle fitted with one or two twenty-five-watt bulbs. Most detrimental to the healing process in such cases is the local application of medication or ointments. Hot soaks are absolutely forbidden.

In sum, the categorical association of diabetes and amputation is totally unfair. The well-regulated diabetic should not sustain any nerve damage whatsoever, and so should not incur foot lesions. Where such damage has occurred, it is still possible to avoid serious foot lesions with proper foot hygiene and podiatry. And even in those cases where such lesions do exist or infection arises, complete healing can be obtained by the application of appropriate treatment.

Other medical complications

Patients who become overapprehensive about diabetes and the complications described above also tend to invent connections to all kinds of other illnesses.

For instance, B.J., a well-controlled, well-adjusted diabetic, appeared at my office one morning before regular office hours. He had just been discharged from the hospital with a probable recurrence of a malignancy of the colon which had been resected one year previously. He was receiving radiotherapy for this condition.

Two nights before he had experienced a burning sensation of the tongue and found he was urinating at night every hour and a half to two hours. He interpreted this symptom as being identical to those he had had at the onset of his diabetes and became fearful that his diabetes was out of kilter. Based on all he had heard from other diabetics, he even deduced that his body chemistry had been deranged by the X-ray treatments! The fact is that his symptoms were indicative of something else entirely and that his diabetes had remained perfectly controlled; in fact it tested even better than it had six weeks before. His concern was needless at a time when the best possible attitude was of vital importance.

Recently, I received a telephone call from the daughter of a seventy-seven-year-old man who had had to have his leg amputed, and then nearly died from a pulmonary embolism. He had diabetes, but his operation had nothing to do with it. Nevertheless, when his daughter heard about it, she became greatly alarmed, and even though I explained that her father's diabetes was very mild and would not harm him in the least, my words did little to calm her fears. Because of the scare stories she'd heard, she became almost as concerned about the diabetes as about her father's amputation and embolism—to absolutely no point, except to worry herself without purpose.

Similarly, a patient I know recently returned from the Mayo Clinic following removal of a brain tumor and a subsequent prostate operation. He had lost a lot of weight, but was getting better, and one would imagine that his wife, a registered nurse, would have rejoiced at his recovery. Instead, she became greatly perturbed by the belief that her husband's increased food intake, necessary to gain weight, was going to aggravate his diabetes! The diabetes was actually very mild and had been readily controlled without medication throughout the various hospital procedures to which he had been subjected. Still, her concern took up valuable time and energy.

At the root of this overemphasis on diabetes and other illnesses, especially in the hospital, is the opinion discussed near the opening of this chapter that the control of diabetes is deranged by any illness. The *fact* is, the majority of diabetic patients who are admitted to the hospital with another illness have been under treatment by their physician for some length of time and have attained at least fairly good control. To be well-controlled it is not always possible, or at all necessary, to have a normal blood sugar and a sugar-free urine at all times. The well-controlled patient, whose blood sugar is "normally" elevated with a moderate amount of sugar in the urine, should have no difficulties whatsoever recovering from other diseases or surgery.

As a matter of fact, it is difficult for me to recall any instances of patients whose diabetes control went awry following heart attacks, infections or surgical procedures as long as there was no lapse in their regular prehospital treatment of drugs, insulin and diet. The diabetic should have no undue fear of other illness or operations.

The same is true of the other complications we have discussed in this chapter. The important thing to remember is that though the diabetic can be privy to a number of complications, many of these are just as likely for the *nondiabetic* as for the diabetic, and none of these are present except in a relatively small minority of cases. With the proper care, as recommended here and by a knowledgeable physician, these complications, should they arise, can be kept to a minimum, and with the medical technology now available, even most of those cases can be or will shortly be controlled. Don't let that cry of "Fire!" frighten you.

7

DIABETES IN CHILDREN

FORTUNATELY, DIABETES is not a common occurrence among children (less than five percent of recognized diabetics are under fifteen years of age), but when it does occur, it poses very special problems in terms of diabetic neurosis.

Obviously, any continuing illness in children carries with it great emotional stress, both for the child and for the family, and this is especially true in the case of diabetes. The onset of the disease in a teenage boy or girl, for example, can be a traumatic event; it may be very difficult for the teenager to cope with the knowledge that he has a disease, that he must remain a diabetic for the rest of his life.

"Why me?" he asks, especially when he is informed that his whole life-style may have to be restricted—what he does, what he eats, where he goes. He may churn up deep feelings of guilt and search his past to discover what sin he has committed to deserve such "punishment." In an effort to hide or overcome such guilt feelings, he may begin challenging society or blaming others, especially his parents, for his becoming a diabetic. Worst of all, he may reject the disease entirely. Emotionally immature, still unsure of his identity, he may refuse to accept the reality of his medical situation and neglect his daily insulin injections or fail to follow his doctor's advice.

He may also use the disease as an excuse—a way

to avoid school or undesired competition and work —or, consciously or unconsciously, as a weapon. How many other children have such a powerful weapon to invoke against parents, teachers or society in general? To get his way or show his displeasure, he need only refuse to eat.

For the older child, college and its life-style raise additional problems. Decisions concerning such common occurrences as drinking, for instance, can be difficult and, at a time when the adolescent wishes to emulate his peers, he is constantly reminded that he is different: that he must undergo daily insulin injections and restrictions on diet, that he must make special preparations for unexpected exercise, that he must guard against hypoglycemia. Even the usual ID bracelet must never obscure the disc which states, "I am a diabetic."

Parental concern, although of quite a different nature, is just as strong. The following remarks, from a father who discovered that his child had diabetes, is typical:

"The doctor must have been looking at us rather closely as my wife and I sat in his office expecting the worst, and then hearing our suspicions clearly confirmed. I'm sure that neither of us knew exactly what we were thinking at that moment, for it was a jolt . . . We had thought this might be the case but had desperately hoped it would not be. Now, suddenly. we had this totally new situation on our hands which neither of us was ready, willing or able to cope with.

"Of course, the doctor (who had delivered all four of our sons) was trying to assure us that the end of the world had not yet arrived and Larry could live a normal life. Our family doctor had never deceived us, and I suppose this should have been enough to allay our fears, but it wasn't. It didn't even begin to untie the anxious knot in the pit of my stomach.

"After the initial shock wore off and I began to

use more reason and less emotion, I learned that the local hospital was giving a course in the basics of diabetes for the benefit of juvenile diabetics and, more important, for their parents.

"At the first meeting, I thought I'd confused the room numbers and was at a session of Alcoholics Anonymous. It was awful. One of the first things the doctor asked of that rather shy group in attendance was 'How many of you are diabetics?' Just as straight out as that! I watched my twelve-year-old son rather timidly raise his hand to about half-mast and mentally countered: 'What a way to start a class on diabetes.'

"Then it really hit me—not only because my son had diabetes, and I was scared silly as to how he would make out in school all by himself, but also because I had been teaching for almost thirty years, and I didn't have the foggiest idea what I would, could or even should do if one of my students had an insulin reaction. If I didn't know, how many other teachers would?"[1]

Fearful parents augment the emotional problems of their diabetic child in ways both subtle and overt. The cycle often begins when someone attempts to establish whether heredity can explain the reason for the child's disease. Though the only familial line may be old Uncle John who had diabetes when he died at age eighty-two, this remote connection is sufficient to supply a source for guilt.

Another and closer source of guilt comes when the mother is questioned about her pregnancy. She becomes convinced that she must have made errors, especially in her diet, while carrying the child, and now tries to redeem herself by constant and excessively careful surveillance of the child's meals. As her diabetic offspring becomes the focus of attention, desserts for all family members begin to disappear, life becomes more regimented, and family closeness often disintegrates. Hostilities that had been dormant suddenly emerge like swarming termites.

Nor is the family's peace of mind improved by information gleaned from other diabetics or even from "expert" commentary printed in various publications. The following statement from a Cleveland newspaper was made by the president of a local chapter of the National Juvenile Diabetic Foundation, an organization charged with the responsibility of *improving* the lot of diabetic children and their parents:

"They get their children up in the morning, give them insulin shots, see them off to school with their tags in place, their special candy in their pockets.

"The candy is not a treat. It is meant to save the child's life if the body chemistry goes awry.

"The tags are not jewelry. They are worn to alert a stranger who could find the child in insulin shock.

"For the mother of the diabetic child, life is a constant worry, a constant watching for telltale signs of trouble.

"She knows it is important for him to lead as normal a life as possible, but she knows also that there is a tragic difference between her child and the child next door.

"Yet, when diabetes is found in a child, the reaction on the part of friends and relatives is usually: 'Just be thankful that it is not a serious disease.'

" 'What could be more serious?' asks Mrs. George Hawk, president of the local chapter of the National Juvenile Diabetes Foundation, and the mother of a four-year-old diabetic. 'Our children usually live only twenty-seven years after the disease is discovered in them. They face blindness, severe kidney damage, the loss of their legs.'

"Diabetes is the fifth leading cause of death in the country."[2]

Imagine the parents of a diabetic child, without any other information about diabetes to offset it, reading such a news item! The damage to family morale caused by such totally unwarranted, unbalanced articles is all too obvious.

PREMATURE AGING LINKED TO DIABETES

This alarming headline, printed in a Cleveland, Ohio, daily newspaper,[3] is another example of the type of writing that can be so injurious to the diabetic child and his family. The news item was based on an article by Dr. Robert H. Kohn, professor of pathology at Case Western Reserve University Medical School. Dr. Kohn stated that severe diabetes starting in childhood may cause an accelerated aging of important connective tissue in the body, making the young old before their time; and he described connective tissue resembling tissue of people aged eighty-four and one hundred and six in patients whose actual ages were thirty-three and forty-four.

Such an article should never have been printed, for Dr. Kohn acknowledges that the three diabetic cases were only a small part of a long-term study of aging, that they were inconclusive and did not prove that the described changes were the result of diabetes. The fact of the matter is, nondiabetic persons *also* experience the greatest increase in stiffness of the connective tissue between the ages of thirty and fifty.

The list of such misleading published statements goes on and on. Consider this statement in the *American Medical News* by Dr. Arthur Rubinstein:

Diabetes, though "manageable" in most adult victims, takes on a grimmer aspect when it strikes children. Though the one-million-plus juvenile diabetics can buy time with insulin and regular care, there is no tangible hope of a cure or a way to head off the more serious complications in later life.

Young diabetics should be told the truth. It's self-defeating not to in the long run, since for the time being there isn't a thing we can do about it.[4]

Very well, let us tell young diabetics the facts. But is this bleak, depressing picture really the truth?

With optimal or adequate treatment, diabetes need not disable children nor hinder their activity in any way. The children grow normally, attend school, get married and raise families like anyone else. They are able to attend college and participate in athletics and other college activities. Upon completion of schooling, they hold positions in keeping with their abilities, and they live to an age comparable to that of other healthy children.

These are the facts. But the key to all of it is proper treatment. Let's look now at the diabetic child, see how his diabetes differs from that of most adults and how this diabetes can best be treated.

Insulin

Insulin is almost always essential to the control of diabetes in children. Even if, as sometimes happens, there is a brief period of remission when insulin could be discontinued, the physician is wise to continue at least "token" injections during this period. Dr. Stuart Carne explains why:

In a very few children, there may be a period usually shortly after the initial diagnosis has been made, when control of the diabetes appears to be satisfactory without insulin, but almost always this "honeymoon" period is brief and the need for insulin soon reappears. It is, therefore, unfair in such cases to discontinue the insulin, however little the quantity needed, because the psychological trauma of having to resume injections may be worse than the advantage of temporarily stopping them.

There are extremely few children (perhaps only a handful recorded in the world medical literature) with proven diabetes in whom there is any lengthy period of freedom from the need for insulin.[5]

In other words, once the child has adjusted to the idea of daily injections, halting them—since this would almost certainly be only temporary—would give the child unwarranted reason to believe his diabetes was improving, that he might never need the injections again. The return to the injections could be traumatic.

Diabetes in children is characterized by marked rises and sudden precipitous drops in blood sugar—changes which range from perhaps 70 mg. percent to 500 mg. percent. Because of such major fluctuations, the diabetic child is more prone than most diabetic adults to hypoglycemia (insulin reaction), and should be taught to recognize the symptoms—declining academic performance, unusual fatigue, lack of concentration, inattention, behavioral problems—and to overcome them quickly by eating something. The child's teacher should also be alert to the symptoms and bring them promptly to the attention of the school nurse and the parents.

Hypoglycemia can be treated by administering sugar in one of many forms. If the child is awake and cooperative, he can be given several small sugar cubes or fruit juice with added sugar (a glass of orange juice with one or two tablespoons of sugar), carbonated beverages (not diet colas) or candy, and the symptoms should clear in ten or fifteen minutes.

If the child is irrational, combative, semiconscious, or unconscious, don't attempt to force fluids. Take him to the nearest hospital emergency room where intravenous glucose or glucagon can be administered.

Most important of all, however, care should be taken to stop hypoglycemia before it starts. Dr. G. D. Molnar[6] stresses that insulin overdosage is the most significant cause of hypoglycemia in the young diabetic —and as we have seen, this overdosage is very often the result of mistaken attempts to achieve and maintain sugar-free urines. Such attempts are not only unrealistic but dangerous. For the best diabetic control, it is frequently essential to compromise the strict blood sugar standards many doctors have promulgated. "In some patients," Dr. H. C. Knowles points out, "you have to tolerate high sugar levels." Another diabetes expert, Dr. R. F. Bradley, readily admits that some sugar is often acceptable and realistic treatment.[7]

Multiple doses (rather than a single daily injection) may also be helpful in avoiding insulin reaction. At least three diabetic authorities agree that the most successful treatment of a juvenile diabetic is obtained this way.[8] Dr. Molnar, for example, suggests that one daily injection of intermediate-acting insulin should be tried first, then mixtures, then up to as many as four doses of short-acting insulin. This last regimen may be difficult for many schedules, but it does have the advantage of stimulating the action of the normal pancreas and permitting the lowest possible total dose of insulin.

Over the years, I have found the most effective arrangement for the large majority of young diabetic patients to be two doses of insulin rather than the single dose prescribed most commonly. At first, I start diabetic patients on regular insulin because its effect is more predictable, but I usually find it necessary later to add an intermediate-acting insulin (Lente, Globin or NPH) to one or both doses.

Whatever the method, one fact stands out: Every diabetic has an individual insulin dosage which is best for him. It is the physician's responsibility to find this dosage and carefully tailor his prescription to the patient's special requirements.

Before we leave the subject of insulin, one last word about the child's responsibility. Since insulin is a major factor in the treatment of his diabetes, it is very important that the child be instructed by his physician in the use of insulin soon after the disease is diagnosed, even if the child is too young yet to give himself the injections. He should learn about the insulin's importance to the body, the proper method of administration, the amount and type to give, and where to inject it. By the time they are ten years old, many children are able to properly administer insulin to themselves.

Diet and exercise

The young person with diabetes faces many challenges, but also possesses the same basic requirements, both physical and emotional, that we all share. His diet, for example, must be designed to meet all his needs for growth, maturation and the varying energy outbursts of childhood. In most cases, the school lunch program is acceptable for the noon meal.

The most important thing to remember is that the energy value of the overall diet must be designed so that the child can attain and then maintain an ideal body weight. In fact, his diet will be so well balanced that the entire family could take note of it. A family with a diabetic child often finds that its nutrition is *improved* after it adopts the basic pattern recommended for the patient!

As for sports, there is no reason why a diabetic child should be kept from physical activity or participation in athletic programs—over ninety-five percent of the diabetic patients in one study could and did participate fully in all the school and extracurricular activities they wanted to. It should always be borne in mind, however, that, as with the omission of a meal, strenuous activity without additional food can induce hypoglycemia, so children with diabetes must always have food readily available. They should eat before and, if necessary, during competition, and they must be taught to recognize their responses to unusual physical exertion. The school should cooperate in allowing the child to eat his snack whenever and wherever it is needed—at his desk, for example.

The recommended approach

The child who becomes angry and frustrated because he has diabetes is responding in a very normal manner. He must be made to realize that he will not become ill from his diabetes if he follows instructions, and his family must avoid treating him as if he were an invalid. He will then come to realize that he is not so different from anyone else, including his peers.

He should be told the complete truth about his diabetes. Since he will be assuming the responsibility for his care when he is old enough, it is essential that he fully understand and accept his condition. *It is no more rational to be secretive or untruthful about diabetes than it is to withhold information about tonsillitis, asthma or a broken leg.*

Everyone around the child should assist him to grow emotionally, to accept the responsibility for his own care, to look forward to his future with a positive attitude. Teachers and other school personnel should be made to understand that they can make a very important contribution to this area, and should be taught about the child's condition, the potential problems that may occur during school hours and the physician's specific recommendations as they relate to school.

Drs. Alexander Marble, Priscilla White, Jean-

Philippe Assal and Donal B. Martin present the very best kind of approach in their excellent chapters in *Counseling and Rehabilitating the Diabetic.*[9] They treat the whole child rather than just the disease, viewing a normal life as their therapeutic goal, stressing the need to stimulate "self-confidence and independence" as well as to acquire discipline. They encourage confidentiality, availability and understanding in order to offset the sense of isolation and "difference" that often comes with diabetes in the young.

Because of the severe emotional impact of the appearance of diabetes on the child's parents, I always devote many hours at the outset to conferences with all the immediate family members. Even though they are often crushed, confused and emotionally drained when they contemplate the future of their child, most of them eventually respond well to an honest approach and become emotionally adjusted to the situation. It is absolutely necessary to continue the discussions, though. Many parents need a great deal of support.

The adolescent himself welcomes complete honesty and nonjudgmental discussions with his physician. Given the right kind of guidance, his diabetes can even be a positive impetus toward growth and maturity. A frank, objective talk by a doctor who is not emotionally involved with the family can eliminate many of the fantasies the child may have, fantasies promoted by the parents' guilt and their need to conceal their feelings. The physician should explain to both the child and the family the history of the disease and its misapprehensions: that its cause is unknown; that the symptoms result from an insulin deficiency—and that with insulin available, the disorder can be overcome so that the body functions normally.

The fear of severe dietary restrictions can be forgotten. Today's diabetic child is permitted all the food other children eat, and he grows like anyone else. In order to achieve all this, however, there is one inconvenience: regular visits to the doctor's office so that the physician can observe the diabetes closely and maintain the best possible control.

Dr. E. Podell summarizes very well the proper approach to diabetes in children:

1. Establish goals based on reality, not fantasy.
2. Provide total education about diabetes. The young diabetic must be familiar with every aspect of diabetes, and the educational process should include results of the latest research.
3. Establish self-responsibility as soon as possible. This should go beyond simply the self-administration of insulin and should also include the responsibility for purchasing and caring for his insulin and syringes.
4. Provide an adult figure, who is not involved with the child's everyday life, to whom he can relate. The physician can certainly be this person, and his support and counseling can greatly enhance the adolescent's emotional stability. The physician needs to establish confidentiality and still be able to involve the total family when conflicts are related to parent-child relationships.
5. Recognize the importance of the child's peer relationships. Healthy friendships (and antagonisms) allow the diabetic adolescent to work out mood swings and identify their causes.
6. Consider the realities of the frequent change in his life-style. *Change* is one word that can be used universally to describe the world of the adolescent.[10]

A great deal of credit is due the mother and father who are forthright with their child about his thoughts and assist in his learning to accept diabetes. The diabetic child who makes a good adjustment reflects the healthy attitudes of his parents, and a child is fortunate if his parents support him well and learn to handle their own concerns in this matter. The discipline he learns at home will help to develop a mature, responsible person who will be able to take pride in his ability to manage his own health problems successfully.

Overprotection

Even the most well-intentioned parents find it difficult to avoid displaying at least some measure of overprotectiveness toward the diabetic child. In addition, the very idea of "being sick" can make some children feel less capable than their friends, so special efforts should be made to develop their sense of independence.

I particularly recommend the use of camps for diabetics, whenever they are available. As R. K. McGraw and L. B. Travis found when they evaluated a group of children with Diabetes Mellitus before and after attending a special camp, those who attended showed a significant increase in their self-esteem and a heartening decrease in anxiety.[11]

One example is Wilderness Adventure, a two-and-one-half-week program offered to thirty diabetic teenagers by the Indiana Diabetes Association. Designed to teach them self-reliance, the trip takes them from Indiana to a Boy Scout camp in northern Wisconsin where they maintain their own camp and cook their meals outdoors. They even take a five-day canoe trip on the Manakagon River, a project which might once have posed a threat to diabetics, but is now made possible, according to camp director Dr. Sam M. Wentworth, by the availability and variety of light, easily transportable freeze-dried foods, which provide the essential nutrients needed to meet their diet requirements. Also included in the camping adventure is a day-long "swamp hike." The words "I can't" are not permitted, says Dr. Wentworth, unless the youngsters try first. "All too often in real life," he adds, "a large number of teenagers defeat themselves before tackling something."[12]

Another example is a Colorado diabetic camp program, in which a group of eleven- and twelve-year-old diabetic boys proved, by reaching the top of a 13,000-foot peak, that they could, within reason, do anything other youngsters could do. "Diabetic children are often overprotected," said Dr. William A. Schneider, medical director of the camp conducted by the Colorado Diabetes Association. "We wanted them to have the experience of being a person out in the wilds of Colorado."[13]

The opportunities afforded by special diabetic camps are well summarized by the father of an actual case:

"I believe that my wife and I had a feeling somewhat akin to Hannibal at the crest of the Alps when we sent Larry to camp for a week last summer. He sailed through one week of activities without a problem, all on his own without help from anyone! This was a direct result of the training he received, and it taught him more about the fact that a diabetic can and should follow a normal life than anything he could read or hear."[14]

8

RESEARCH

RESEARCH PROGRAMS currently underway and likely to bear fruit within the next few years offer more reasons for a positive attitude by the diabetic and his family.

In May 1973 a group of self-proclaimed "militant" parents met in Philadelphia and chartered the Juvenile Diabetes Foundation to gather funds for research and put lobbying pressure on Congress to increase government appropriations. Ninety percent of what they raise goes directly to research, and, along with other important organizations such as the American Diabetes Association, their efforts were instrumental in the passage and enactment of a program providing ninety-four million dollars for better health, a substantial portion of which has gone specifically to diabetes research.

On June 23, 1973, the featured speaker at the annual banquet of the American Diabetes Association in Chicago was Dr. G. Donald Whedon, director of the National Institute of Arthritis, Metabolism and Digestive Disease. He described some of the diabetes-related activities of his agency, which included one hundred thirteen research grants, counting fellowships and training grants, costing the Institute a total of $6.4 million for extramural diabetes research and research-training support. He stressed the remarkable increase in research this evidenced and the hope it held for the future—and today such hope is even stronger, as many of these and other research programs begin to bear results. Progress can be seen in a multitude of areas, such as prevention of diabetes, improved diagnostic technique, better effectiveness for insulin, simpler techniques for the delivery of insulin, improved monitoring of blood sugar, artificial pancreas and transplantation of the pancreas islets which supply insulin. The work being done in these areas is very complex, but the following is a brief overview:

Prevention

There is mounting evidence from animal experimentation that viruses disrupt the release of insulin or kill the insulin-producing cells entirely. Dr. E. J. Rayfield of Frederick, Maryland, inoculated hamsters with encephalitis virus and found that the invading virus killed some of the beta cells which produce insulin, and that the hamsters subsequently developed diabetes. After the infection subsided, the insulin content in the serum remained lower than before the infection, leaving the impression that diabetes may develop as a result of viral infection.

In addition, statistical evidence suggests that mumps, German measles and some influenza-like viruses may trigger diabetes in genetically prone youngsters.

The significance of this research is immense. If diabetes is the result of a virus, and if the diabetic virus or viruses in humans can be identified—then an anti-diabetes vaccine can be made.

Diagnosis

A test that measures insulin in humans may be better than the conventional glucose-tolerance test to detect the presence of diabetes. For the past few years, Chicago pathologist Dr. Joseph Kraft has comparison-tested a new insulin test with the conventional glucose tolerance test on some three thousand patients at St. Joseph's Hospital. The results: nearly half of the fifteen hundred patients whose blood sugar registered normal on the conventional blood sugar test showed "diabetic patterns" on the new insulin test. This may help considerably with early warning.

Improving insulin effectiveness

The addition of a human growth hormone antagonist (a hormone that inhibits the secretion of other hormones) offers very good prospects for enhancing the post-meal effect of insulin. Dr. Roger Guillemin of the Salk Institute in San Diego has synthesized such a hormone (somatostatin) from the hypothalamus of the brain. In a recent study of six juvenile diabetics at the University of California in San Francisco, it was found that a single injection combining insulin and somatostatin proved more effective than insulin alone in abolishing post-meal hyperglycemia in diabetic patients.

"The most interesting and most stimulating aspect for the future," commented Dr. Guillemin, "is that the simultaneous administration of somatostatin and regular insulin produces dramatic decreases of blood sugar . . . [it holds out] much encouragement for the future in the treatment of juvenile diabetes."[1]

Insulin delivery

Dr. John Urquhart and Nancy Keller of Palo Alto, California, have shown that insulin can pass from a reservoir outside a large vein directly through the vein's walls (presumably by diffusion) into the blood at therapeutically useful rates. This development, especially when considered with the possibility of transplanting insulin-producing cells, presents great potential as a possible alternative to injection.

Experiments now in progress indicate that another delivery system may be produced by way of liposomes, tiny cell-like structures which were discovered in 1964. Thanks to work by Dr. Gerald Weisman and Dr. Grazia Sissa completed in 1970, it is now possible to fill these microscopically small structures with insulin. Early tests indicate that the insulin-filled liposomes, taken orally, will slip past the digestive juices without being destroyed and, like tiny Trojan horses, deliver their insulin into the system.

Monitoring the system

At present, diabetic patients can tell when their blood sugar levels are high only by measuring spill-over in the urine. To better monitor the blood sugar, Dr. Stuart J. Soeldner has developed an implanted "glucose sensor," a dime-shaped disc that generates small electric currents in reaction to changing glucose levels. Dr. Soeldner wired the sensor to an implanted, matchbook-size radio transmitter in rats and rabbits, with effective results. He has also implanted the sensor in monkeys and kept it there for as long as four months with no rejection problem. "Assuming there are no hitches in further monkey tests," says Dr. Soeldner, "clinical trials can soon be underway."[2]

In a human, the sensor system would probably be implanted in the abdominal area, its attached transmitter signaling to a radio receiver on the belt of the diabetic. Every fifteen minutes, the receiver dial would indicate the blood sugar level, and if it went too high or too low, a "bleeper" would sound a warning.

Several steps must be taken before the glucose sensor can be ready for human implantation, however. Experiments are underway now to test the sensor by using it to monitor blood at the bedside of hospital patients. With it, monitoring can be carried out constantly with less than 2 ml. of blood per hour. This type of experiment, aside from improving the technique of sensor implantation, is directly beneficial to the patient. It permits doctors to be better informed of the progress of therapy, helps them to apply appropriate treatment without the delay of running blood samples through a clinical laboratory and spares the patient the inconvenience of multiple blood sampling.

The next step will be the complete control of the diabetic using the unit *outside* the body. When the patient is fully "tuned" to his or her unit, the final step can be undertaken: implantation.

Artificial pancreas

Eventually, rather than simply warning the patients of excessive blood sugar levels, such sensors as are mentioned above might be connected directly to computers. Already, Miles Laboratory has incorporated the entire device—sensor, autoanalyzer, computer and typewriter—into a single portable module about the size of a television set, an apparatus that monitors blood sugar levels and dispenses insulin or glucose as required. Such units have already been put into use in Toronto and Ulm, Germany, laboratories.[3,4] Tested on dogs for several years before being used to treat human patients, the human studies culminated nine years of work by a team under the medical direction of Dr. Bernard S. Leibel, associate professor of medicine at the University of Toronto's Banting and Best Department of Medical Research.

A working model of another artificial pancreas

capable of releasing insulin in response to the body's changing needs has been developed by Dr. Samuel Bessman and colleagues at the University of Southern California.[5] It is a closed loop control system built around three sub-systems: the patient, the pumping and autoanalyzing apparatus and the computer.

It has now become feasible due to the development of two devices—a stable implantable sensor able to measure tissue fluid glucose, and a tiny pump sensitive enough to pump against any possible changes in internal pressure and efficient enough to utilize a very small power supply. The rest of the technology—the micro-computer, tissue-compatible plastic case and miniature power supply—all come from other medical advances such as the cardiac pacemaker.

The volume of the entire apparatus is only about the size of an egg. It works like this: a tiny sensor under the skin, about the size of a thumbnail, receives about twenty-five to thirty microliters of blood per minute from a vein in front of the elbow. The blood goes into a modified chemical analyzer in which the blood sugar level is determined, then the signal is automatically fed into a computer which compares it to the "normal" figures stored in its memory. The computer then adjusts any deviations from the norm by controlling the insulin or glucose pumps.

The pump responds with graded numbers of strokes to signals generated by the miniature computer circuit. Its power supply, equal to one-sixth of the power now used for the cardiac pacemaker, can function under optimum conditions for more than eight years, pumping at the rate of one hundred divided doses per day.

This new device has proved able to maintain normoglycemia in diabetics under all conditions studied, the results showing an unprecedented degree of control. Patients require about *one-third* their usual subcutaneous dose of insulin.

Dr. A. Michael Albisser, professor of medical engineering at the University of Toronto, has estimated, however, that it will take several years before development of a fully miniaturized, implantable artificial pancreas will be ready for clinical trial.

Pancreas transplant

The first success with the transplant of a pancreas was reported in 1963 by DeJode and Howard, who showed that it was possible to reverse diabetes by means of a graft of a whole pancreas. By the end of 1970, twenty-three pancreatic transplants had been performed throughout the world. Unfortunately, however, the successes were short-lived. Although some of the grafts "took," and hyperglycemia was satisfactorily reduced for a time, all patients died of various causes, the longest surviving somewhat over a year.

One problem encountered in transplanting the whole pancreas is the disposition of the digestive juices. A technique has now been developed for channeling these juices into the urinary bladder via the ureter, and in two instances has been carried out successfully in conjunction with kidney transplantation performed at a different time.

The basic problem with transplanting the entire pancreas is summarized very succinctly by Dr. Ricketts: "The success of immunology has not advanced far enough to guarantee against rejection."[6]

But if progress in this area has been somewhat disappointing, the strides made in the next area more than offset it.

Transplantation of cells

Researchers have turned to another substitute for the ailing pancreas: the transplantation of insulin-producing *cells* rather than an entire organ. Such experiments have been successfully carried out with rats by the late Dr. Arnold Lazarow of the University of Minnesota, and the result has held down blood sugar levels and allowed the rats to gain weight.[7]

Dr. Lazarow obtained the clumps of cells from fetal pancreas, grew them in cultures and then transplanted them to the diabetic host, where the beta cells functioned normally. Although here too, cells, like the total pancreas, may be rejected by the host, experimentation thus far indicates that cells grown in organ cultures are less likely to be rejected.

In general

The pieces of the research jigsaw puzzle needed to find the cure for diabetes are slowly being found and put together. Thanks to increased talent and financial support, the past few years have seen a definite acceleration in the pace with which we are acquiring new knowledge, and with continued efforts on the part of fine organizations like the Juvenile Diabetes Association, we can expect a research "explosion" very soon.

There is no doubt that the discovery of the cause and cure for diabetes is near at hand—the knowledge needed to make this dramatic breakthrough is accumulating at this very moment.

9

THE POSITIVE
APPROACH

PROPER DIABETIC EDUCATION is essential if one is to understand and be able to ignore the scare stories told, the exaggerated articles and books written, the TV shows broadcast about diabetes. Only through such education can diabetics and their families avoid or overcome diabetic neurosis, and only in this way can they develop the affirmative approach so vital to proper care and treatment of the disease.

Diabetes is best controlled not by fear and dread, but by knowledge and self-assurance—by a positive attitude.

The advantages of such an attitude may become clear through this example. In the course of my medical practice, I have encountered many patients with insomnia. Most tend to complain about their sleeplessness, about the fact that they are unable to enjoy the same amount of rest as other members of their household, but others (I recall one in particular) have turned the disability to their advantage instead of bemoaning it. Recognizing that for some unexplained reason they simply can't sleep as long as most people, they take those hours—hours of solitude—and use them to gain extra knowledge. One car company executive told me quite frankly that he considered his insomnia to be "the secret of my success."

In much the same way, diabetes can be one's "secret

of success" in terms of a healthy, happier life. If patients accept the reality of the disease rather than fight it, and use it as a barometric enforcer of good health, they will find themselves turning a negative into a positive.

Dr. L. Matthews, professor of pediatrics at Case Western Reserve University, who we first met in Chapter One, expresses this very well:

> So you have diabetes. Is that so bad? I don't think so, and I feel I should know since I've had diabetes since 1957. If one had a choice, I'm certain we would all choose perfect health. But if one has to have a chronic disease, and we really have no choice, then I feel we are fortunate to have diabetes.
>
> I found it possible to achieve every goal I set for myself in academic pediatrics, to raise a family of five energetic children, to paint my own home, to wallpaper every room of it, to be a family traveler and camper, and even extend the lives of my cystic fibrosis patients, some of whom have diabetes in addition to cystic fibrosis.
>
> I write this only to attempt to convince you that having diabetes can even be an advantage. It's a disease you don't have to be ashamed of, one you can even be proud to have conquered. Don't hide it or use it as an excuse. Use it as an increased incentive.[1]

E. Hill, a diabetic of many years, presents much the same viewpoint:

> When someone asks what kind of problems I have with diabetes, I usually reply that the only problem I have is in thinking of a problem when asked. Having reached the age of twenty-three after twenty-one years of diabetes, my life is as active

and full as that of any of my fraternity chums
who have a reputation of being the most active
students at the dental school.

My diabetes has not prevented me from achiev-
ing everything I have wanted to accomplish, and
I see no reason for that condition to change.[2]

Children can be taught such a positive attitude at
a very early age. Danny R., a nine-year-old diabetic,
has been under my care for two years. From the start,
his parents accepted the disease properly, and the
youngster had no trepidation whatsoever about his diabetes. Last summer he attended an overnight camp for
two weeks. This was not a camp for diabetics; accordingly, Danny had to administer his own insulin
and eat the regular camp food. The result: a wonder-
ful time. As one might expect, Danny returned home
in the best of health and spirits and with a renewed
sense of self-assurance.

Recently, the father of two teen-age diabetic sisters,
who had received their diagnoses within two weeks of
each other, phoned to inquire about a minor ailment
one of them had. During the conversation, he expressed
his appreciation for the services given his daughters.
He pointed out that following their diagnoses, they
had walked around completely bewildered, their heads
bowed, but after receiving a clearer, more compre-
hensive picture of their disease and their future lives,
they had perked up rapidly and become two normal,
happy girls.

This kind of positive acceptance can be used as an
example for adults as well. A thirty-year-old woman
who was unable to accept the fact of her diabetes was
counseled by a young nurse who had had diabetes
since the age of nine. She pointed out that if a nine-
year-old child and her family could adjust themselves
to accept diabetes—sufficiently so as to raise that
child and send her happily into a nursing career—then

why couldn't a mature, thirty-year-old woman make the same sort of adjustment? The woman made an about-face in her attitude.

The positive thoughts that pass through the minds of well-adjusted diabetics are best expressed in the words of the patients themselves. Here, for example, is Bill Talbert's story of his youth:

I was ten years old when my illness began. I would come home from school and plop into bed, almost too tired to raise my head. I gulped down water as if I were marooned on a desert island. I ate as if food was going to be outlawed. I went to the bathroom too often.

My mother and father took me to the doctor. I had diabetes. Not too many years before, there was nothing for a diabetic to do but waste away and ultimately die. The discovery of insulin brightened the overall picture, but the diabetic's fate was inactivity. Baseball was out. No more sports of any kind for me—until that day Dad came home with a package under his arm.

"What's that?" my mother asked.

"A tennis racket for Billy," said my father.

My mother was visibly upset. "You're not going to let that boy play tennis?" she inquired, incredulous.

I was 14 then. My dreams of baseball dashed, I was happy to play any sport—even a sissy game like tennis.[8]

Bill Talbert did play that "sissy" game. He went on to become one of the world's best-known tennis champions, winning such titles as the National Men's Doubles Championship 1942, 1945, 1946, 1948; the Clay Court Singles 1945; the National Men's Indoor Doubles 1949, 1950, 1951, 1954; and the National Men's Indoor Singles 1948 and 1951.

Today, Bill Talbert is a very successful executive for the Security-Columbian Banknote Company of New York.

Ron Santo, the noted baseball player, found out he was a diabetic when he was just nineteen years old. He says:

> When you consider all the diseases that can't be controlled, it's almost a relief to have diabetes. I eat just about anything I want. I haven't had any complications. I've had operations and injuries— my jaw busted, a broken wrist, cuts—and they all healed well because I have taken very good care of myself. I've never been in a coma.
>
> For the first five years I had diabetes, I pretty much kept it to myself. But after I made a couple of All-Star games and felt I was becoming established, I told the club's team physician, Dr. Jacob Suker, and the organization. Even then I kept it quiet for a while, but now I make a point of talking to groups of kids who are diabetics, and to their parents. I try to give them my side of the story, which is, "Sure diabetes is a disease, but it's a disease you can handle if you just make an effort."
>
> My life is no different from anybody else's. The shot to me is nothing. It's my normal routine— like waking up and putting on my pants. It's not a disease you can take lightly, and if you don't accept it, you are going to have problems. But if you know what it's all about, you can live a full, healthy life.[4]

Bruce Taylor is not a celebrity—at least not yet— but the words of this young aspiring writer seem appropriate here:

> One day I learned that a friend of my father's had cancer of the stomach. Knowing that I was a

diabetic, he said that he would give anything if he could have an injection every day to control his disease. What he said punctured my balloon of self-pity. I realized that if it were not for insulin, I would be dead.

Before insulin was first discovered by Drs. Banting and Best, I would have been put on a starvation diet and had a life expectancy of a few months to—at most—a few years. I began to see how lucky I was after all those days when I had simply accepted life, never giving a thought as to how beautifully such a complex machine as the human body works.

Insulin. That one word is now synonymous with life. Now every day that I am able to live is indeed a special day. I keep thinking whenever I hear of someone with cancer, "What would he give if he could have an injection a day that would alleviate his disease so that he could lead a normal life?"

What would you give if you were blind and found that by taking an injection each day you could see? What would you give? Or ask yourself what can one give for all the courage, time, energy, experiments, failures, successes which some people face so that someone else may live—someone like me, whom Dr. Banting and Dr. Best never met or ever will meet?

Thanks. I worship life. Every minute. When I became diabetic and then realized how lucky I was to still be alive, I began to see how incredibly beautiful the world is. From then on, whenever I saw a wave kiss the shore or watched a sunset, my reaction was no longer, "Gee, isn't that nice." Instead, it was, "My God! I'm alive to see this!"

And when I saw a person suffering, I no longer said, "Gee, that's too bad," but rather, "What can I do to help?" That's why I worked for my degree in sociology from the University of Washington. And that's why I have begun to write. Perhaps there is something I can do or say that will help others. Perhaps these words have given someone, somewhere, something that he or she did not have before. It may be hope, for that is what I feel— hope and faith in the future. Hope and faith in humanity. The nobility of mankind seeking answers, never satisfied—striving, conquering, healing.

No, no. I will not be resentful of diabetes again. I have learned too much. I have learned not only how beautiful life is but what it means to live. I have learned how to make every minute count, how to regard every flower as a universe within itself, how to regard life as a universe.

That is what diabetes has taught me. It has caused a new awareness in my life. Although being a diabetic has its complications, the fact that I live—that I have life—far outweighs any detrimental factor.

Now I know how valuable life is.[5]

As I reach the end of this book, it seems fitting to return to the beginning—to the words of Mary Tyler Moore, one of television's most talented and successful actresses.[6]

"The most amazing thing about diabetes," said Ms. Moore, "is the complete lack of knowledge that exists about it. When I first learned I had it, I was very frightened. I wondered, 'Am I going to be an invalid? Will I be bedridden?' I just didn't know."

But Mary Tyler Moore went on to find out. She learned about diabetes—learned how to care for it and how to make it work for her.

"I check in with my doctor much more than the average person does," the actress explains. "He can spot trouble in other areas long before the average person is going to spot it because the average person might go to his doctor only once or twice a year. I go at least four or five times a year."

Finally, Ms. Moore offers some words of inspiration for all diabetics and their families: "Maybe it isn't a blessing to be a diabetic, but a person who finds out they have diabetes can easily turn what might appear to be a negative into a very important positive. I know that I did."

And you can, too.

NOTES AND REFERENCES

Chapter One: Fiction Versus Fact

NOTES
1. *Wall Street Journal,* November 4, 1974.
2. *Diabetes Forecast,* July-August 1976.
3. Winsted, M.: "New Weapons Against a Major Killer," *Arizona Republic,* September, 1974.
4. Matthews, L.: "Life with Diabetes," *Diabetes Newsletter,* Diabetes Association of Greater Cleveland, 12:2 (April), 1974.

Chapter Two: Basic Questions and Answers

NOTES
1. Boshell, B. R.: "Fellow Diabetic Is Best Teacher About Regimen," *Int. Med. News,* 7:1, No. 10 (May 15), 1974.
2. Schnatz, J. D.: "Self-Care Instruction Reduces Need to Hospitalize Diabetics," *Int. Med. News,* 7:45, No. 17 (Sept. 1), 1974.
3. Duncan, T. G.: "Advance for Diabetics—U-100 Insulin Improves Therapy," *Chronic Disease,* 8:1 (Nov.), 1974.
4. Davidson, J. A.; Galloway, J. A.; Petersen, B. H.; Wentworth, S. M.; and Crabtree, R. E.: "Purified

Insulins Seen Alleviating Allergies," *Chronic Disease, 8:*1 (Dec.), 1974.

5. Service, F. J. and Molnar, G. D.: "On the Nature of Diabetes and the Need for Urine Testing," *ADA Forecast, 27:*12 (March-April), 1974.

6. Forsham, P.: "Improved Treatment for Diabetes Outlined," *Chronic Disease, 7:*1, No. 11 (Nov.), 1973.

7. Siperstein, M. D.: "Insulin and the Juvenile Diabetic," *Diabetology '74.* Report from the Geigy Symposium, Albuquerque, New Mexico.

8. Sims, E. A. and Sims, D. F.: "A Dialogue about Diabetes and Exercise," *ADA Forecast, 27:*27–31 (Sept.-Oct.), 1974.

OTHER REFERENCES

• Podoll, M.: "Life Style Conflict of the Adolescent Diabetic," *Medical Insight,* pp. 21-26 (March), 1974.

• Marble, A.: "Oral Agents Revisited," *Diabetes Forecast, 27:*2–6 (Nov.-Dec.), 1974.

• Horwitz, N.: "FDA Makes Big Concessions on Oral Antidiabetic Labeling," *Medical Tribune* (March 27), 1974.

• Bourne, H.: "UGDP Results Are 'Irrelevant' in Some Cases," *Int. Med. News, 7:*4, No. 8 (April 15), 1974.

Chapter Three: Keeping Control

NOTES

1. Service, F. J. and Molnar, G. D.: "On the Nature of Diabetes and the Need for Urine Testing," *ADA Forecast* (March-April), 1974.

2. Feldman, J. M. and Lebovitz, F. L.: "Test for Glycosuria: An Analysis of Factors that Cause Misleading Results," *Diabetes* (Feb.), 1973.

3, 5. Gastineau, C. F.: "Ask Me Another," *ADA Forecast* (March-April), 1973.

4. Burrington, J. S.: "Burrington Cites Clinitest Tablets' Peril to Children," *Medical Tribune* (March 12), 1975.

6. Molnar, G. D., Taylor, W. F. and Ho, M. M.: "Day to Day Variation of Continuously Monitored Glycemia: A Further Measure of Diabetic Instability," *Diabetologia,* 1972.

7. Sadler, H.: *Int. Med. News* (April), 1973.

Chapter Four: Food and Drink

NOTES

1, 2, 5, 6. West, K. M.: "Diet Therapy of Diabetes: An Analysis of Failure," *Ann. Int. Med., 79:*425–434 (Sept.), 1973.

3. French, J. B.: "Diabetics Get Dietetic Boost," p. 1C, *The Cleveland Plain Dealer,* Oct. 26, 1974.

4. Brunzell, J. D.; Lerner, R. L.; Prote, D., Jr.; and Bierman, E. L.: "Effect of a Fat Free, High Carbohydrate Diet on Diabetic Subjects with Fasting Hyperglycemia," *Diabetes, 23:*138–142 (Feb.), 1974.

7. Davidoff, F. F.: *Medical Opinion, 3:*24–30 (June), 1974.

OTHER REFERENCES

• Sussman, K. E.: "The Elderly Patient's Diet," *Consultant, 13:*165–174 (Sept.), 1974.

• Weinsier, R. L.; Seeman, Ann; Herrera, G.; Assal, G. P.; Soeldner, J. S.; and Gleason, R. E.: "High-and-Low-Carbohydrate Diets in Diabetes Mellitus: Study on Effects on Diabetic Control, Insulin Secretion, and Blood Lipids," *Ann. Int. Med., 80:*332–334 (March), 1974.

• Lestradet, H.; Dartois, A. M.; and Machinot, S.:

"Spontaneous Food Intake in Children and Juvenile Diabetics Treated with Insulin," *Excerpta Medica, No. 280*:127 (July), 1973.

- Shuman, C. R.: "Using Steroids in Diabetes," *Chronic Disease, 8*:1 (Nov.), 1974.

Chapter Five: Marriage and Children

NOTES

1. Beck, P.: "Women with Severe Diabetes Advised to Avoid Pregnancy," *Medical Tribune,* p. 29 (Oct. 17), 1973.
2. "Managing Common Complications in the Newborn," article in *Patient Care,* p. 24 (July 1), 1974.
3. Tyson, J. E.; Khojandi, M.; and Tsai, A. Y. M.: "Diabetic's Diet Control Key to Normal Birth," *Medical Tribune, 15*:3 (Feb. 20), 1974.
4. Rimoin, D. L.: "Many Faceted Diabetes is 'A Geneticist's Nightmare' ": *Ob. Gyn. News,* p. 20, May 1, 1973.
5. Pyke, D. A.: "Diabetes May Not Be Genetic," *Dimensions, 2*:1 (Nov.), 1973.
6. Neel, J. V.: "Explaining the Genetics Nightmare of Diabetes to Your Patients," *Medical Opinion, 2*: 58–68 (Oct.), 1973.

OTHER REFERENCES

- Gruenwald, L.; Simpson, N. E.; and Fraser, F. C.: "Genetic Counseling in Diabetes Mellitus, Questions and Answers," *JAMA, 230*:468, Oct. 21, 1974.
- Schwaninger, D.: "Follow-Up of Children Born to Diabetic Mothers," *Schweiz Med. Wochenschr, 103*: 1130–1133 (Aug. 11), 1973.
- Srongin, L. M.: "The Miracle," *ADA Forecast,* pp. 25–27 (June-July), 1974.

Chapter Six: Complications

NOTES

1. Critique of *Counseling and Rehabilitating the Diabetic,* John Cull and Richard Hardy; C. C. Thomas, 1974 (Dolger and Dolger), *ADA Forecast, 27*:13 (Nov.-Dec.), 1974.
2. Siperstein, M. D.: "Aging and Basement Membranes," *Diabetology '74,* Report from Geigy Symposium, Albuquerque, New Mexico.
3. Black, M. B.; Berk, J. E.; Fridlander, L. S.; Steiner, D. F.; and Rubinstein, A. H.: "Diabetic Ketoacidosis Associated with Mumps Infection: Occurrence in a Patient with Macromylasemia," *Ann. Int. Med., 78*:663–669 (May), 1973.
4. Ricketts, H. T. (Acting Editor): "The University Group Diabetes Program—A Study of the Effects of Hypoglycemia Agents on Vascular Complications in Patients with Adult-Onset Diabetes; Part I—Design, Methods and Baseline Results," *Diabetes, 19:* 747–783 (Supplement, 1970) and "Part II—Mortality Results," *Diabetes, 19*:787–830 (Supplement, 1970).

More unhelpful scare stories regarding heart disease were made in a recent announcement by the University Group Diabetes Program, which unsettled the equanimity of the diabetic population at large and those taking oral antidiabetic drugs in particular. According to the UGDP study, deaths from cardiovascular disease were twice as frequent among diabetics treated with tolbutamide (Orinase) than among those treated by diet alone or with insulin.

As a result, the Food and Drug Administration was impelled to issue grave warnings as to the potential hazards of the oral antidiabetic drugs, and statements to this effect were incorporated in the package inserts. This statistical data created a great deal of confusion and uncertainty in the medical profession. In fact, the therapeutic zeal to control diabetes (of such vast importance to all diabetics) was shaken by the claim that long-term use of a drug like tolbutamide might hasten the development of arterial lesions. If this well-researched drug is unsafe, doctors and patients reasoned, what about many other drugs?

These reactions on the part of doctors and diabetics are particularly hard to take in light of the statement by Dr. Fajans, professor of internal medicine in the Division of Endocrinology and Metabolism and the Metabolic Research Unit, University of Michigan School, Ann Arbor, who said:

"No other study has confirmed the UGDP results. It is very difficult for me to say the UGDP has proven that these drugs are harmful. I'm hard pressed to say that I can truly believe increased risk has been demonstrated."

Moreover, a fourteen-year study at Ann Arbor of young latent diabetics and controls has not shown tolbutamide to be associated with an increased prevalence of heart abnormalities.

The UGDP study succeeded overwhelmingly in only one respect: upsetting the happiness of thousands of diabetics who may have felt quite secure in their day-to-day living only to be told that they were in danger of dropping dead momentarily with a heart attack. One thing is certain: a very long period of time will be required to heal the emotional trauma inflicted by the UGDP study.

5. Moss, J. M.: "Current Opinion: Open Letter to *Washington Post*," Medical Tribune, p. 7 (Nov. 13), 1974.
6. Moss, J. M. and Delawter, D.: "Georgetown Study Disputes UGDP Findings," *Int. Med. News*, p. 14 (Oct. 1), 1973.

7. Kupfer, C.: "Evaluation of the Treatment of Diabetic Retinopathy: A Research Project," *The Sight-Saving Review*, pp. 17-28 (Spring), 1973.

8. O'Grady, G.: "Surgery Offers Hope in Diabetic Retinopathy," *Int. Med. News*, 7:23 (Aug.), 1974.

9. Reinecke, R. D.: "New Procedure Aids Diabetic Blind," *Chronic Disease*, 8:23 (Dec.), 1974.

10. Ellison, J.: "Eye Surgery Aids Blinded Area Diabetic," *Cleveland Plain Dealer*, Oct. 9, 1974.

11. Kussman, M., 35 al.: "Early Grafts Urged for Diabetics with Nephropathy," *Medical Tribune*, 15:10, No. 27 (July), 1974.

12. Hampers, C.: "Diabetics Should Not Be Refused Chronic Dialysis," *Int. Med. News*, 7:1 (Sept), 1974.

OTHER REFERENCES

• *1972 Annual Report*, American Diabetes Association.

• "Diabetes as the Patient Sees It," *Patient Care*, pp. 21–75 (March 15), 1973.

• Groom, D.: "Diabetes and Heart Disease, Cardiovascular Review," *Medical World News*, pp. 15–16, 1973.

• Drury, I. M. and Timoney, F. J.: "Oral Hypoglycemic Agents and Cardiovascular Deaths in Diabetes," *Acta Diabetologica Latina*, 9:245 (July-Aug.), 1972.

• Miller, L. V. and Goldstein, J.: "A Dissent from the Conclusions of the UGDP Study," *Personal Communication*.

• Rubin, W., ed.: "Who Evaluates Drugs?" *Int. Med. News*, 7:1 (Nov. 1), 1974.

• Kahn, O.; Wagner, W.; and Bessman, A. N.: "Mortality of Diabetic Patients Treated Surgically for Lower Limb Infection and for Gangrene," *Diabetes*, 23:287–292 (April), 1974.

Chapter Seven: Diabetes in Children

NOTES
1. Harris, W. M.: "Teaching the Teacher," *ADA Forecast,* 27:30–32 (Nov.-Dec.), 1974.
2. Vincent, B.: "Juvenile Diabetes: A Tragic Difference in Children," *The Cleveland Press,* May 22, 1974.
3. Ellison, J.: "Premature Aging Linked to Diabetes," The *Cleveland Plain Dealer* (July 6), 1974.
4. Rubinstein, A.: "Diabetics' Parents Form Foundation," *American Medical News,* p. 8 (Feb. 18), 1974.
5. Carne, Stuart: "How They Treat Diabetes in Children," *Resident and Staff Physician* (July), 1976.
6, 7, 8. Baker, L.; Bradley, R. F.; Molnar, G. D.; and Knowles, H. C., Jr.: "Emotions Called Factor in Instability of Brittle Diabetic," *Int. Med. News, 7:* 30–31 (June 1), 1974.
9. Critique of *Counseling and Rehabilitating the Diabetic* (Dolger and Dolger), *ADA Forecast,* 27:13 (Nov.-Dec.), 1974.
10. Podoll, E.: "Life Style Conflict of the Adolescent Diabetic," *Medical Insight,* pp. 21–26 (March), 1974.
11. McGraw, R. K. and Travis L. B.: "Psychological Effects of a Special Summer Camp on Juvenile Diabetics," *Diabetes, 22:*275–279 (April), 1973.
12. Wentworth, S. M.: "Diabetic Teens Adventure in Wisconsin Wilderness," *Affiliate Builder, No. 18:*7 (Sept.-Oct.), 1973.
13. Schneider, W. A.: "Boys Climb Colorado Peak," *Affiliate Builder, No. 18:*7–8 (Sept.-Oct.), 1973.
14. Harris, W. M.: "Teaching the Teacher," *ADA Forecast,* 27:30–32 (Nov.-Dec.), 1974.

Chapter Eight: Research

NOTES
1. Guillemin, R.: "Somatostatin in Insulin Shot Enhances Post-Meal Effect," *Medical Tribune, 15*:1 (Dec. 4), 1974.
2. *Wall Street Journal,* November 7, 1974, p. 1.
3. Albisser, A. M., et al.: "Use of Artificial Pancreas to Treat Diabetes," *Int. Med. News, 7*:1 and 25 (July 15), 1974.
4. Albisser, A. M.: "Computerized Artificial Pancreas Passes First Clinical Trials," *Medical Tribune, 15*:1 (Oct. 9), 1974.
5. Bessman, S. P.: "Status of the Artificial Beta Cell," *Metabolic Therapy, 3*:1, Winter, 1974.
6. Ricketts, H. T.: "Pancreatic Transplants: New Wrinkles," *JAMA, 228:* 609–610 (April 29), 1974.
7. Lazarow, A.: "Diabetes Investigator Misses Hopes, Caution," *Chronic Disease,* p. 2 (Sept.), 1973.

OTHER REFERENCES
• Rubinstein, Dr. Arthur: *American Medical News* (Feb. 18), 1974.
• Scharp, D. W. et al.: "Implanted Pancreatic Islets Work in Diabetic Primates," *Medical Tribune, 15:* 1, *No. 27* (July 17), 1974.
• Duncan, T. G. and Oppenheimer, H. E.: "New Discoveries in Diabetes Reported," *ADA Forecast, 27:* 15–18 (Sept.-Oct.), 1974.

Chapter Nine: The Positive Approach

NOTES
1. Matthews, L.: "Life with Diabetes," *Diabetes News-*

letter, Diabetes Association of Greater Cleveland, *12:*2 (April), 1974.

2. Hill, E.: "Life with Diabetes," *Diabetes Newsletter,* Diabetes Association of Greater Cleveland, *12:*2 (April), 1974.

3. Talbert, W. F.: "40-Love Is Sweeping the Country!" *Prism,* 8:30–35 (Nov.), 1973.

4. Shaw, J.: "Ron Santo and Diabetes: Accept It, Live a Full Life," *Sportsmedicine,* 2:61–63 (June), 1974.

5. Taylor, Bruce: *ADA Forecast* (June-July), 1973.

6. "Mary Tyler Moore Wins Again," *ADA Forecast,* 27:6 (May-June), 1974.

OTHER REFERENCES

• "A Diabetic 'Famous People List'—Perhaps One Day You!" *Diabetes Newsletter,* Diabetes Association of Greater Cleveland, *11:*2 (August), 1973.

• Flanders, C. E.: "Dick Batchelder—Star Racer and Diabetic," *ADA Forecast,* 27:27–31 (Sept.-Oct.), 1974.

• Sims, E. A. and Sims, D. F.: "A Dialogue about Diabetes and Exercise," *ADA Forecast,* 27:27–31 (Sept.-Oct.), 1974.

• Hsu, T. H.; Paz-Guevara, A. T.; and White, P.: "40-Year Juvenile-Diabetic Patients Do Well," *Medical Tribune, 15:*2 (July 24), 1974.

INDEX

153

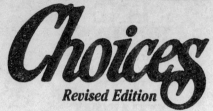